Today is Still the Day

A Blueprint for a 3D Life of Wholeness

Ann Musico, CHHC

REVIEWS

"Today is Still the Day, is a book JAM PACKED with information that will change your life. You think you've read it all concerning health and fitness? I can tell you... this book is revolutionary! Ann has a way of taking complex information and laying it out in a way we can all understand it. Not only is this book motivating, but you'll feel like Ann is your buddy & mentor on the road to health and wellness.

Marcy Travis, Certified Career Coach | Discover Your Best Work Options

"Are you searching for breakthrough, valuable wellness advice that you can really add into your lifestyle? Look no further....Author Ann Musico is a profoundly passionate and loving health coach who gives you a seven week plan in her book Today is Still the Day. The steps provided by Ann are both powerful and incremental so that you can transform your lifestyle with ease and reach your physical, emotional and spiritual goals."

**Dr. Lynne E. Kavulich, Board Certified American Academy of Anti-Aging Board and Clinical Nutrition Author and Speaker.
www.AmericanWellnessCare.com**

"I met Ann Musico through a mutual friend a few years ago, at a time when my life was in great upheaval; after a 30-minute chat with her on the phone, I felt like I had met a friend for life.

Ann is gracious, kind, understanding, and very knowledgeable in her gifted profession. Ann is always learning and growing in the knowledge of nutrition and healing, both physical and emotional. After hearing about her nutritional plan and book, I decided to hire Ann as my nutrition coach. In a very short period of time, not only was I losing weight and feeling better, but my self-confidence and hope for my future was being restored.

Ann thoroughly understands the Spirit, soul, body connection. She guides you through her book with information and steps to take that are doable and not overwhelming so you can be the best you God wants you to be. Small changes do bring big results!

I heartily endorse the use of this book and Ann's nutritional coaching program as the next step on your path to freedom and fruitfulness for your overall health and well-being as a way of life.

Ann Musico, her knowledge, kindness and friendship, is by far one of the greatest gifts the Lord has ever given to me. Be blessed in your journey,

Linda Alan, Accountant, MELT Method Instructor

Ann is an incredible Health Coach! I started with Ann about 5 years ago. I was struggling with my weight. A program I had used for years, no longer worked for me. Ann's plan, taught me how to eat clean; her knowledge of supplements has helped tremendously! I lost 40 pounds and kept it off! I am 54 years old, and the only prescription drug I am on is for my thyroid. I just had complete blood work done. My doctor said it was perfect! I thank Ann for her guidance!

Luanne Begany, Hairdresser

My wife had been receiving coaching from Ann Musico. She would constantly repeat things Ann taught her. Her name was a household name. I was on blood pressure and cholesterol medicine. I had a physical, now my sugar was high! The doctor gave me three months to try to bring it down. Now I finally listened to my wife. I started coaching with Ann. With her help, I not only avoided diabetes medicine but also came off ALL medicine! What a blessing she has been to our family!

Paul Begany, Salesman

If you are searching for a solution to wholeness and regaining your happy healthy life, you have found it in connecting with the author of this book. Ann Musico, within this book, enables you to identify areas where you are struggling and provides realistic helps to free yourself of any roadblocks that are limiting your life. Whether it is weight loss, diabetes, lethargy in life, or just confusion over the myriad of information in the diet and exercise world, this book breaks things down and provides you a plan to follow in achieving your goals. Each chapter provides meaningful yet simple guidelines that you can put into place right now to enhance your life and get to the heart of your concerns. It is encouraging and personal and comes from her heart to help individuals be the best they can be! Everyone will find something valuable in this book that will help he or she make the healthy changes he or she has desired for years. Her experience in helping others just blossoms throughout this book, and each reader will find simple yet effective solutions for his or her everyday health issues.

Lori Yaw

ISBN: 978-0-692-19634-2

DEDICATION

I could do nothing without my incredible and loving Heavenly Father, my Lord Jesus and His precious Holy Spirit. I cannot ever thank You enough for the grace to accomplish what You have put on my heart to do. Truly You are everything to me and all glory and honor belong to You alone.

I am blessed to have my wonderful, supportive husband, Alex, who encourages and supports me in whatever the Lord leads me to do.

I also have three of the most amazing children, Christopher, Matthew and Elizabeth, who are my constant sources of encouragement, motivation and support, daily enriching my life beyond imagining. Along with their spouses, they are my greatest encouragement and cheering section.

I also dedicate this book to all those I hope will find encouragement, support and improved health and wholeness in these pages.

PREFACE

This is an updated version of my original book, Today's the Day. As I have been using the plan with clients and getting feedback from people who've bought the book and done the plan, I have made some changes to simplify it and include new research that I've come across over the last five years. There seems to be new (and often conflicting) information, daily. I like to get down to basics and keep things simple.

Anyone can diet and lose weight. The trick is to lose fat, retrain taste buds, create healthier habits and keep the weight off long-term. You actually do more damage when you yo-yo diet than if you just stayed overweight! Unfortunately, most people who begin a diet, either don't ever reach their goal or if they do, they are unable to maintain it. In my opinion, if you can't sustain the changes and make them part of your daily routine, you won't stick with it, and you will just default to the habits that got you sick and overweight to begin with.

The plan detailed in this book will teach you how to break addictions to processed, sugar-laden foods and create vibrant wholeness – spirit, soul and body. This is more than just a diet. Most diets don't even consider spirit and soul health. You are a spirit who has a soul (a mind, will and emotions) and you live in a physical body. You can't overlook any one of these aspects of your being and expect to be truly healthy in the best sense of that word.

This book will touch on facets of weight loss and fitness "diets" don't such as: why is it important to detox your spirit and soul? How can you nourish them? Why should you? How can you rest and reboot on a daily basis? Why is that even important? Why does your self-talk matter so much? What does any of this have to do with weight loss?

Any diet will cause you to lose weight – temporarily. Making lasting, healthy changes that become part of your new normal is what you want. My hope and prayer is that this will be your blueprint for true wholeness.

Wishing you health and blessings,

Ann Musico

TABLE OF CONTENTS

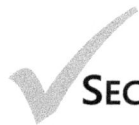

✓ SECTION ONE

BACKGROUND AND BASICS

Before We Get Into It...

If you are familiar with my original book, *Today is the Day 7 Week Fitness Plan*, or my coaching, you know that this is not a "diet" but principles and strategies you can use to upgrade your lifestyle choices in order to create true health and wholeness. It is more than just losing a certain number of pounds or getting to a specific number on the scale. Wholeness encompasses so much more than that.

I am all for getting yourself to a healthy weight where you look and feel your best. It was the reason I developed my plan over 20 years ago for myself. But that shouldn't be the be-all end-all. You'll notice the sub-title of this book is "A Blueprint for a 3D Life of Wholeness." The 3D refers to the three dimensions of our being: spirit, soul (which includes mind, will and emotions) and body. These three dimensions must be in harmony and balance in order for you to enjoy health and wholeness.

In all my coaching, including this plan, there are four keys we apply to each dimension, and those four keys are:

- ✓ Detox/Cleanse
- ✓ Nourish/Fuel
- ✓ Intentional Exertion/Exercise
- ✓ Rest/Reboot

So we cleanse and detox not just our bodies, but also our spirits and souls (mind/thinking, will and emotions). Then we nourish and fuel each properly. Nutrition is more than just food. It encompasses whatever we take into our bodies – spirit, soul and body. That includes beliefs, thoughts and emotions as much as it does protein, carbs and fat.

We intentionally exercise and strengthen each area, and then comes rest/sleep and rebooting, which includes stress management, relaxing, and learning to dream and imagine again.

You can see this is very comprehensive. It is also effective, because when you address each area in this way, you are not just losing a few pounds and then going back to the old habits that got you fat and sick in the first place. You are creating a healthier lifestyle.

A diet is a temporary change. This is intended to be a permanent change. That's why I call it a blueprint, not a diet. I don't believe in "one size fits all." We are all unique and certain foods and nutrients are good for me, but they may not work for you. This is why it is a blueprint. I put in place some foundational principles, but you can adjust any part of it to better address your needs. Nothing is written in stone and you don't have to follow anything exactly.

Don't think you can't enjoy holiday goodies or have some birthday cake. Life is meant to be enjoyed and those things are part of it. Think about restructuring your habits so that 80-90% of the time you are sticking to your healthy choices. The 10 or 20% of the time you go off and have the Christmas cookies or birthday cake or whatever the particular treat is, it will not ruin all your other efforts. And when you see how much better you feel when you eat properly, you will want to get back to your normal, healthy eating as quickly as possible.

If you want to skip directly to the plan in Section Two, you can do that and then read the rest as you wish to. If you would like daily coaching that supports your efforts through the plan, visit my website and sign up. There are certain supplements I particularly like and recommend. I have provided a link to a page on my website where I will keep those sites updated. You can access it here: http://www.threedimensionalvitality.com/resource-page-for-book.html or https://bit.ly/2Eqo1sb

Unfortunately things change quite often and I hate to have links to products that are no longer offered or broken links. This way you can always either access the information on the Resources page or email me at ann@threedimensionalvitality.com and ask.

* Let me address something right here at the beginning. People have asked me if they must be a Christian to benefit from this plan since I address life and health from my Christian beliefs and they are clearly part of the plan. The short answer is no, you do not. My experience has been that Bible-based Christian principles enhance every aspect of the program. Although you do not have to be a Christian, an open mind is crucial. My personal relationship with Jesus catapulted me to another dimension of existence and I genuinely wish for others to experience the same. However, I have worked with believers and non-believers alike, and the principles are

effective regardless. While I do not force my beliefs on anyone, I do not hide them either.

So, now let's get started....

I Should Already Know This!

Health and weight loss are simple and complicated at the same time. It should be as simple as eating clean, whole foods and staying active, but of course it isn't quite that simple. To begin with, our food supply is contaminated with herbicides, pesticides, hormones, antibiotics and GMOs, and the problem is we have no idea how they will affect us long term.

Life in this day and age is hectic and stressful and there is information overload. We learn some new (usually contradictory) information almost daily. So what do you believe? And what do you do?

So many women I have worked with struggled with whether or not to commit to coaching with me because they said they were ashamed and felt they should already know how to do this. How does anyone really know exactly how to do this unless they are willing to admit they don't know it all?

I was at a loss as to why so many people take the time to do the free consultation and then never respond to my follow up email and never get the information they wanted initially. I had a wonderful consultation with a lovely lady and we discussed the results of her health evaluation and some thoughts about what she was struggling with. During our conversation I mentioned to her that she obviously is doing many things right from her responses, and it could just be some minor "tweaks" I might suggest that could help her see progress.

She admitted that she hesitated doing the evaluation for weeks. I asked why and she said while she was excited to speak to someone and get another perspective on what she was already doing, she also struggled with feelings of fear and shame! It didn't really occur to me that people would feel ashamed asking for help, or afraid of what they may be told – but obviously they do! This is a big reason why I have added *Tapping into Health*, the Christian EFT sessions, to the coaching plan. Guilt, fear and shame only hold you back from being your best self and EFT is a very simple and effective way of addressing those negative emotions.

I assured her that we all need help from time to time – who does it all perfectly or never has a question? No one I know, including myself! We are human beings and God put us in relationship because many times we can see how to help someone else where we are blind to our own needs. But we have to push past those emotions and open ourselves to new ways of seeing and doing things.

Another client so eloquently said, *"We think for some reason we are supposed to have it all together and not need help from anyone. I think that is why so many exercise machines and pills are sold but people are still unhealthy and overweight. You offer your strength and wisdom with love, without judgment. Yes, we all have strengths and weaknesses and you realize that up front with your clients. I appreciate your willingness to note that we ALL fall short (Romans 3:23) and need help!"*

Often times that is exactly when we begin to see things clearly and find the support and encouragement to take those first steps toward achieving our goals. So if fear or shame are holding you back – I urge you to push past them. Let's make forward progress toward your goal!

Why Women Struggle So Much (Can you relate?)

There are myriad reasons why any one person, man or woman, might be struggling with weight loss. There are obvious reasons such as lack of activity, eating too many processed foods, or just eating too much in general. There can be hormonal issues, food intolerances or allergies, interactions with medications and digestive issues. However, that's not all.

As a woman I deal primarily with women, and I see something at work in women of all ages. I have a daughter in her 20s and daughters-in-law in their early 30s. I have worked with young women in their 20s and early 30s. I see them dealing with the stresses of beginning a career, navigating relationships, planning weddings, buying a home, starting a family, and dealing with newborns. Just listing all those things stresses me out! And I've been through it all.

Many are working more than one job or working a full time job and either going to school to finish a degree part time or working a side job. That means often they are rushing from one job to another and usually healthy eating falls by the wayside. Often they are burning the candle at both ends to just get it all done and sleep suffers. Where do they fit in time to exercise? And who has the energy?

Then you have women in their 40s and beyond. While their children may be grown and out of the house, that doesn't mean they are not impacted by whatever is going on in their children's lives. I can personally attest to that. I heard someone say once that a mother is only as happy as her unhappiest child, and that is so true. If one of my children is going through a difficult time, it is as if it is happening to me.

Many women at this time are either re-entering the work force now that children are gone, or are considering making a change, starting a side business, or going part-time. They may be adjusting to a spouse's retirement. They may be experiencing financial crises with these changes. They may also have become caretakers for elderly or ailing parents or relatives. Many have 20-something children who had to return home, and that creates unique stresses all its own.

None of these things is easy and none of them are conducive to weight loss, much less health and peace. We don't often realize how powerfully stress, anxiety, and lack of peace affect our ability to not only be truly healthy, but also to be able to lose excess weight as well as to maintain a healthy weight.

Life is not necessarily easy or smooth all the time – for men or women. We know this. As women we are usually the peacemakers, caretakers, comforters, nurturers, encouragers and support systems for our spouses and families, and this is a huge privilege as well as responsibility. It is nothing new, however. Just read Proverbs 31 and you see this is how God created us as women.

If you see yourself in one of these descriptions and you are struggling to lose weight and find balance in your life, I want to encourage you. Thankfully we go through different seasons in life. For moms with small children, know that this season will go by much more quickly than it seems to when you are in the midst of it. All my coaching addresses spirit, soul and body because health is more than the absence of illness or a certain number on the scale – it is wholeness. It begins, particularly for women, in putting yourself on the list.

That sounds so simple, and truly it is, but it is not always easy. Often things like guilt come into play. We are supposed to put others before ourselves and we've gotten so good at that we can feel guilty asking for help or taking time out for ourselves. But it isn't an "either-or" situation. It is definitely a process. As with all changes we make, taking one baby step at a time usually works best. We don't have to change everything all at once, but we have to commit to making some gradual changes. You will be surprised at how supportive your family will be when you enlist their help in making changes.

Who knows, you may even encourage them to make their own healthy changes. Many of the women I've worked with have had just that happen with their families. When their spouses see the change in their wives, they are open to hearing what they are doing. One coaching client says:

"I just want to take this time to tell you how wonderful this whole process has been for me.

I have learned so much, not only an education in food values, but spiritually, this has been quite a journey. The daily encouragements and food for thought information have left me thinking and re-evaluating myself and the way I have done things for a long time.

I have thoroughly enjoyed each e-mail and tip that you have sent me along the way. This program is truly life changing and spirit-led. I have incorporated many changes and have felt the benefit of the changes and additions to my life. As I have shared different tips with my family, they also are benefiting as well in their lives, too. The mistakes along the way that pop up have been learning experiences for me to better understand the triggers that always pre-requisite a bad meal or a bad day. That in itself is huge!!! Thank you so much, Ann!"

I have been privileged to have quite a few instances where the spouse or young adult children then sought me out because they saw the positive changes.

We are all works in progress, so whether we like it or not, change is our constant. Once you become aware of some things you can do to put yourself on the list, begin slowly incorporating them into your life and enlist your family's help.

High Quality, One Ingredient Foods

The foundation of health is nutrition. This is true from conception to death! What you eat before you get pregnant as well as while you are carrying your child powerfully impacts his or her development. It is equally true that what emotions you experience and beliefs and thoughts you entertain are just as powerful and impactful. That's true for each of us at each stage of life – so nutrition is the foundation, and we build from there.

It's important to understand food is more than just something to fill your belly with. It is information that speaks to us at the cellular level! Dr. Mark Hyman calls it powerful medicine, and I totally agree. When you stop and think that our food supply is extremely compromised and look at the state of our health as a nation, it's not difficult to see the connection.

To keep things as simple as possible *I focus on choosing the highest quality, one-ingredient foods.* What that means is this:

High quality for me equals properly raised/grown food. So for produce that would be organic, locally grown when possible, fresh or frozen.

With animal foods like meat, dairy, poultry, fish, etc., that means grass-fed and finished, free range, wild caught, pasture raised, and organic where appropriate.

If we are what we eat and digest, then we also are what our food ate!!! Does that make sense to you? If you eat conventionally raised meat from cows that were confined to pens, fed GMO grains and not treated humanely, you are getting the result of that. Their meat will have less healthy fats, more stress hormones, and most likely antibiotics and hormones that they were administered. They pass that on to you.

So quality is always first and foremost.

Then what I call one-ingredient foods. These are foods that would "be" ingredients in a packaged food. They *don't have* ingredients – they *are* an ingredient. Examples would be cucumbers, walnuts, chia seeds, peppers, arugula, kale, eggs, beef, lamb, chicken, quinoa, oats, blueberries, celery and avocados.

Hopefully you get the picture. Keep it simple. Look for the highest quality real, whole, fresh or frozen one-ingredient foods you can find or afford and create your meals from there. If that's the only change you make, you will be doing yourself a huge favor and reap a multitude of benefits simply from doing this one thing. I do understand organic and grass-fed are more expensive, but they are worth the extra cost. I have included a link to Environmental Working Group which posts their Dirty Dozen, Clean 15 lists. You don't have to buy everything organic. You can put your zip code into

Local Harvest and find farms, farmers markets, CSAs and more in your local area.

You are What You Eat – Even Spiritually, Mentally and Emotionally!

I've already made it clear, I think, that choosing high quality, real food is the way to properly nourish your physical body. Too many people today are not only overweight and obese but also malnourished. It's true. You can fill your belly and put pounds on and yet be starving your cells of the nutrition they need to be healthy. Again, quality is key!

Often we find ourselves in the habit of eating a certain "junk" food. Think of how often people spend hundreds of dollars a month on those sugary, expensive coffee drinks. We like the taste or the texture and ignore the fact that it is not providing anything that truly nourishes us. But it becomes our habit. Sooner or later we will reap the results of those choices.

The same is true spiritually. There is plenty of "spiritual junk food" readily available. If you choose that, you can become spiritually malnourished. Just as you require more than one meal a week physically, your spirit requires more than just an hour of nourishment on Sundays.

This is true mentally as well. The things you read, watch on TV, listen to and think about will either build you up or tear you down. If you continually watch "junk" on TV or the news 24/7 or replay negative, hurtful things over and over in your mind, you are starving yourself just as if you neglected to eat.

We all have a steady stream of thoughts in our heads. Much of this is not truth. It's not even fact. We make the mistake of believing whatever thoughts go through our heads are our truth. God's Word tells us to take every thought captive. I talk about some ways to do that in the actual Plan so we'll get into this more in Section Three. For now keep in mind that you are a spiritual being made in God's image, and much more than simply the sum of your thoughts. We are to have no master other than God and that includes our thoughts. We don't know how to direct our own steps, so we are to be led by the Holy Spirit. We can renew our minds so that all our thoughts can align with His will and Word.

The spiritual and mental nourishment you provide will impact your emotional health. It is all intertwined. Your thoughts will affect your emotions. Your spiritual health will impact your mental and physical health. So it is not enough just to eat a clean diet that nourishes your physical body. That's just one aspect of true nourishment.

Philippians 4:8 in The Passion Translation says it beautifully: *"So keep your thoughts continually fixed on all that is authentic and real, honorable and admirable, beautiful and respectful, pure and holy, merciful and kind. And fasten your thoughts on every glorious work of God, praising him always."*

While I am talking about quality, let's not overlook quality of life! True health is not just the absence of illness. It encompasses spirit, soul (mind, will, emotions) and body. Wholeness more correctly expresses what I mean by health. For me, quality of life is the ability to do the things that bring you joy, to spend time with your family, play with your children or grandchildren, travel, fulfill God's call on your life in whatever unique way He leads you.

The Truth About Calories

"Eat less and exercise more and you'll lose weight."

How often have you read or heard that? Thousands of times most likely. And I'm sure like most people you are thinking – if only it was that easy! But is it true?

This is related to the previous chapter in that it has to do with the quality of your food.

Can you eat 1,000 calories a day of chocolate cake and potato chips, hit the gym for an hour and still lose weight? Are those 1,000 calories going to affect your body the same way 1,000 calories of grass-fed beef and Brussels sprouts would?

Are 160 calories of almonds going to impact your body in the same way as 160 calories of a sugary soda or a candy bar?

You probably already know the answer to those questions is a resounding "No!" Honestly, a calorie is not a calorie! While they're equal by definition in terms of their energy content, your body processes each in a specific way, and these differences have serious implications for weight management.

Let's take it one step further. Even if you eat 1,000 calories of junk food, can you exercise enough to burn it all off and end up losing weight anyway?

Again, that just doesn't work, so the answer is "No." The truth is you can't out-train a bad diet, but you can eat your way to a fitter and healthier body.

The point is this: *the source of the calories is far more important than the amount*, since they are not all metabolized equally.

The food you eat is not just energy but information that literally controls just about every function of your body, including hormones, appetite, brain chemistry, immune system, gene expression, and microbiome with every morsel. And the quality and composition of the information matters more than the quantity. It is similar to programming a computer – garbage in, garbage out!

Calories from carbohydrates (sugars, starchy carbs and grains) raise levels of the storage hormone, insulin and are stored as body fat. Healthy fats, which are the most efficient fuel for your body, and clean protein (think grass-fed, free range, wild caught) have very little impact on your insulin and so help you lose weight.

All these years we have been urged to eat low fat, diet foods, replacing real foods like meat, eggs and avocados with low fat, sugary carb snack foods, exercise like fiends and stick to a certain number of calories and where has it gotten us? Overweight, obese, and in many cases malnourished, diabetic and suffering from heart disease and cancer. Not a very pretty picture.

Remember, I said I like to keep things simple and basic. I tell clients to choose real, whole, high quality one-ingredient foods, eliminate (for the most part), or at the very least, limit grains, sugar and other starchy carbs, replacing them with non-starchy veggies to give you fiber and healthy carbs.

Pay more attention to the quality of your food and the breakdown of the macronutrients (protein, carbs and fats) than the number of calories.

Dr. Mercola says: "*Carbohydrate intake is the primary factor that determines your body's fat ratio, and processed grains and sugars (particularly fructose) are the primary culprits behind our skyrocketing obesity and diabetes rates.*"

Is that all there is to it? Not quite – there are certainly some details we tweak, including hydration, supplements (to be sure you are covering your nutritional bases), inflammation, type and amount of exercise, adequate sleep, hormonal imbalances, stress and self-sabotaging beliefs, meal timing, food allergies and sensitivities, among others.

There's no "one size fits all" answer just as there is no "magic pill." I truly wish there was. But when we use common sense and get back to basics, it's almost amazing to see how well our bodies respond.

Water and Salt – Why?

A foundational principle in this Plan is drinking adequate water. The formula I have used for years is one-half your body weight in ounces with ¼ teaspoon of natural, unprocessed salt like Himalayan Crystal or Celtic Sea, for every 32 ounces which I learned from Dr. Fereydoon Batmanghelidj's books.

People often have no qualms about replacing empty liquid calories with clean water, but they often question why they should include the salt. You don't have to put the salt directly into your water but you can. I do. I have many clients who think that sounds crazy, but after they try it, they just love the energy they get and end up liking the taste as well. You certainly can just measure out the right amount of salt for your water and include it in your food if you prefer.

Let me talk a bit about why the salt is such an important part of this. As with food, the quality is the key. There is a huge difference between processed table salt and natural, unprocessed salt like Himalayan Crystal salt.

Table salt has been stripped of its naturally-occurring minerals during processing. Before I say any more about this, I have to highlight the importance of minerals. According to two-time Nobel Prize winner, Dr. Linus Pauling, *"You can trace every sickness, every disease, and every ailment to a mineral deficiency."* Minerals are the foundation of sound nutrition and health. Without them, no other system in the body works as it should. Amino acids and enzymes don't work when you lack vital minerals, and then vitamins and other nutrients do not get broken down or absorbed. Now back to processed table salt.

Rock salt, which is inferior quality, is mined from the earth and dried at very high temperatures. This high heat changes the chemical structure into sodium chloride. What is left after that process is essentially dead, so synthetic chemical additives are put back in: bleach, to make the salt white, and anti-caking agents to make it pour easily.

Those naturally-occurring minerals that have been stripped away are a critical part of balancing blood pressure, which is why consuming table salt elevates blood pressure. Natural, unprocessed salt is never perfectly white due to its mineral content. It contains more than 80 trace minerals which provide important nutrition to your body. It provides numerous benefits, not the least of which is proper hydration. You can't effectively lose weight or even process emotions if you are dehydrated.

Consuming water with natural salt allows your body to absorb and use the water you are taking in. If you simply drink a lot of water without salt, you will spend a lot of time in the bathroom and that water will not properly hydrate you. It will just pass through you. When you drink too much plain water without the proper concentration of salt, your extracellular fluid (the fluid outside and around your cells) becomes over-diluted. This actually puts extra strain on your body, creates a stress response and slows metabolism – the opposite of what you want.

So don't be afraid of salt as long as it is natural and unprocessed.

Making Friends with Fat

First of all, let's make an important distinction. Healthy, dietary fat is not the same as the cosmetic fat that forms the extra belly fat or saddle bags on your thighs. I think that may be part of why just talking about fat scares people! We've been so indoctrinated to believe that fat is bad and makes you fat that even considering some fat healthy is a stretch for many people.

Fat is one of the three macronutrients your body needs daily. As with everything else, quality is the key here. In case you are not familiar with the macronutrients, they are fat, protein and carbohydrates. Obviously, choosing the best quality of each is going to make or break your diet. Eliminating bad fats like trans-fats or partially hydrogenated and processed vegetable oils like canola, corn, soybean, sunflower, cottonseed and safflower is step one. These are refined, damaged oils which are highly inflammatory to your body. The one exception to this is a trans-fat called CLA: conjugated linoleic acid, which is found naturally in grass-fed dairy and meat. It can actually help you burn fat and is being researched for its cancer and heart protective abilities.

Because it is often the most misunderstood, I wanted to highlight healthy fat. We all know protein is important for building muscle as well as for healthy skin, hair and nails. Choosing the right carbs is also critically important. In reality, you can live without carbs but not fat. You can't live without protein, fat, and water, but you would be just fine without carbs because your body can actually create its own glucose. While I recommend keeping to a low carb diet, I never advocate totally eliminating any macronutrient. Just choose the best quality.

What is healthy fat?

Omega-3 fats, EPA and DHA from cod liver and krill oil and fatty fish like salmon and sardines and nuts like walnuts provide healthy, anti-inflammatory fats. Omega-3 and Omega-6 fatty acids are considered "essential" because your body needs them but can't make them. You must get them from your diet. Because processed foods contain Omega-6 fats, we tend to have too much of these and they can then become inflammatory. Correcting the ratio of Omega-3s to Omega-6 fats is something we must keep in mind to reduce inflammation. Experts have long believed the ratio should be 1:1. People eating a typical Western diet get a ratio of about 15:1, or more Omega-6 to Omega-3.

Omega-9 fats are described as "non-essential," because our bodies can synthesize them from other things we eat, and we don't have to depend on direct dietary sources to obtain them. Omega-9 fats are also known as monounsaturated fats or oleic acid, primarily found in olive oil, olives, avocados, sesame, avocado and almond oil, pistachios, cashews, hazelnuts and macadamia nuts. They have many benefits including heart health, brain health and increased energy.

Saturated fats like pasture butter, ghee, coconut oil, full fat, grass-fed dairy, cheese and meat are another type of healthy fat. These are all good sources of clean energy and necessary for you to be able to absorb fat soluble vitamins like vitamin A, D, E and K.

Eating fat will help your food become more nutritious, which will help your body perform at its highest level. Certain foods you eat, carrots for example, are best cooked whole and eaten with a form a healthy fat in order to absorb all the carotenes and other vitamins they contain that are fat soluble.

A diet rich in healthy fats increases levels of HDL or "good" cholesterol. Higher HDL levels help you produce more growth hormone, which increases the production of amino acids. Clean protein and healthy fat are necessary to build muscle which keeps you strong and helps you lose weight.

Every cell membrane in your body is made of fat and protein. When you include adequate healthy fats in your meals, you feel satiated and not constantly hungry.

So instead of trying to go low calorie or low or no fat – consider including healthy fat, along with clean protein and non-starchy, vegetable carbs and you have the building blocks of a very healthy diet and the backbone of this plan!

Just a quick note about saturated fats and heart disease: we've been told for years that saturated fat causes high cholesterol and heart disease. While I won't get into the details here, suffice it to say it has now been proven that healthy saturated fats do not cause heart disease and do not raise "bad" cholesterol. Sugar and grains increase LDL or bad cholesterol.

http://articles.mercola.com/sites/articles/archive/2014/05/06/saturated-fat-phobia.aspx

Make healthy fat your new best friend. You won't regret it.

What the Heck is Resistant Starch?

There is something called resistant starch (RS) that many are unaware of. Resistant starch is a carb that resists digestion. Where most starches convert to glucose in the small intestine, as other carbohydrates do, RS resists digestion and passes through to the large intestine where it acts much like dietary fiber and is fermented by gut bacteria. So it acts as a prebiotic, feeding the good bacteria in your gut.

This alone is a wonderful thing! These good bacteria improve the absorption of minerals and make it more difficult for the bad bacteria to thrive. RS seems to decrease after meal glucose and insulin response, improve insulin sensitivity, cholesterol, boost metabolism, increase satiety and reduce fat storage. All great things!

Some sources of RS are cooked, cooled and reheated rice, oats or potatoes; beans and legumes, particularly adzuki beans; one to two tablespoons of raw potato starch* daily added into yogurt or a smoothie; and green bananas as well as green banana flour. By the way, baking potatoes seems to increase their RS; baby potatoes are highest in RS, and if you choose to boil your potatoes, use bone broth or stock and then use that liquid in your cooking so you get benefit of all the nutrients!

*Start slowly! Use ¼ teaspoon and work your way up as it can constipate you.

I learned how to include RS with a low carb diet to accomplish the "subsequent meal" effect. It's fascinating. RS blunts insulin and glucose spikes and helps escort the excess sugar out of your body. If you plan a higher carb dinner – maybe a birthday party or dinner out – whatever it may be, research shows if you have resistant starch at the low carb meal *before* the high carb meal, your after-meal, or postprandial glycemic response (PPGR), is improved at the next meal! (The high carb one.)

So if you have a low carb dinner tonight, it helps you at that meal *and* your PPGR will be improved at breakfast tomorrow, especially if it is a higher carb meal, since it is the subsequent meal. It seems to lower the glycemic effect. The low carb meal makes you more carb tolerant at the next meal a handy thing to know.

You can use these hacks whenever you know you'll be having a higher carb meal and include resistant starch with a low carb diet to accomplish the same thing. Bottom line: if you're planning on going higher carb for a meal — for whatever reason — low carb the meal prior to it and/or include RS.

By stabilizing insulin and glucose levels you not only protect yourself from their damaging effects, you also help your body to protect itself from illness by boosting immune function and increasing nutrient absorption, particularly minerals.

You Can Have a Problem with Any Food – Even "Healthy" Food

So many things can come into play when choosing the healthiest diet for you: gender, age, lifestyle, origin, climate, genes, health status and unique toxic load, among other things. Our nutritional requirements vary because we are each unique. In fact, your nutritional requirements will vary over time as well. What works for you at 20 may not be best at 40.

There's all sorts of research proving being a vegetarian, vegan, going paleo, eating keto – you name it – is the "best" and healthiest way to eat. But regardless of what any research says, you must take your own uniqueness into consideration. Any of those diet plans may be good for certain people, but it doesn't mean it is right for you. And even if it is right for you today, it may not be in a year!

Just as "one size fits all" clothing doesn't usually fit everyone well, one size fits all diets don't work for everyone either. What is most important is to know yourself and your make up. Keep it simple. Employ a few basic principles. I spoke earlier about choosing clean, whole, properly raised/grown one-ingredient foods. That's a basic principle. Another is testing specific foods to see if they are causing an inflammatory response in your body. Particularly if it is a food you especially love and eat daily, I would suggest testing.

Foods have an amazing ability to support digestion, heal the 'gut', strengthen immunity, fight infection, reduce inflammation, enhance mood, calm the nervous system, build muscle, boost IQ, alkalinize the body and much more. However, even a healthy food might not agree with your make up at any given time. But how can you know? Kinesiology, or muscle testing, is a very effective way to test which specific foods and even supplements are best for you.

I read about another relatively simple way to test any food you think may be causing problems for you.

Here are the steps to test:

1. Choose a particular food you are going to test and set aside 15-20 minutes where you can just relax. Surfing the net, reading or watching television work well for this test.

2. Take your resting heart rate and write it down.

(You can simply find your pulse with two fingers on the side of your neck or if you have a smart phone, you can download a free heart rate app. Count the beats for 15 seconds and multiply by four for your resting heart rate.)

3. Eat some of the food you are testing. It is best to choose a specific food so you know exactly which food is causing an inflammatory response. If you test a meal you wouldn't know which specific food it is.

4. Remain seated, avoiding anything that would cause a rise in heart rate for 15-20 minutes.

5. Take your resting heart rate again and write this number down.

Here's how to measure the results:

If your heart rate stayed the same after eating the food being tested, then this food most likely does not cause an inflammatory reaction in your body.

If you had a five beat per minute increase, this suggests a small inflammatory response and would be worth retesting to see if it was a fluke or if you indeed have some mild reactivity to that food.

A 10 beat per minute increase clearly shows an inflammatory response to that food and bears keeping track. You would want to avoid this food until you get some indication of why this food is causing this inflammatory response.

An increase greater than 10 suggests a strong reaction and would be wise to avoid this food until you have addressed any underlying digestive issues.

The way this simple test works is this:

1. When we consume a food, it first goes into the stomach for digestion then down into the small intestine to be absorbed. Food particles begin to pass through the small intestine and are absorbed into the bloodstream. As the food particles are absorbed, they come into contact with our white blood cells, the front line of our immune system.

2. As our immune system engages with the food, the white blood cells determine if this food is good for us or a problem. If the food in question is good for us, our immune system doesn't sound the alarm. However, if our immune system has identified this food as problematic, white blood cells will send out messengers to stimulate the immune response (aka inflammatory response).

One of these messengers is called interleukin-6 (IL-6).

3. IL-6 is a pro-inflammatory cytokine, a messenger which alerts the whole immune system to respond because there's something that needs to be defended against. One of the primary ways our immune system responds to an alert is to inflame the area in order to restrict 'the invader' from moving around and causing problems in other parts of the body.

4. When IL-6 is released, it stimulates the sympathetic nervous system (fight or flight) which raises your heart rate.

This is why testing your heart rate before and after a meal can offer profound feedback as to whether your system has identified a specific food as troublesome for your body.

Keep in mind, just because your body may be reactive to a certain food today doesn't mean you have to avoid that food forever. Other factors, like the state of health of your small intestine and whether your immune system is activated, also play important roles in this scenario.

If, however, your heart rate goes up after eating a specific food consistently, it may be best to avoid that food for a sustained period of time in order to give your body a break from the chronic inflammatory response it provokes. It's also helpful to retest soon after just to confirm that the rise in heart rate was actually from eating the food in question.

Mitochondria and Microbiome: Two Words You Must Understand

You may have seen these words in articles and posts recently and wondered what they are and whether you should care. I will not get into a deep explanation. Dr. Mercola and Dr. Hyman both have excellent books and you can find links to them on the resource page on my website. These are two key functions we need to understand and nurture in order to be truly healthy.

Let's begin with mitochondria.

For our purposes here, the simple, basic definition of mitochondria is this: they are tiny power plants in every cell that turn your food and oxygen into energy in the form of ATP via biochemical reactions in your cells. In fact, they produce 90% of the energy generated in your body. And since everything that happens in your body requires energy, keeping the mitochondria healthy impacts everything.

When mitochondria aren't working properly, your body and brain are not working optimally so you may feel more tired and perhaps not as sharp mentally. You'll age more quickly. Mitochondria also play a role in many age-related diseases, such as heart disease, diabetes, and neurodegenerative diseases like Alzheimer's, Parkinson's and ALS. So I think you can see that they are hugely important. So how do you nourish them?

First of all, they like fat! Mitochondria function best when fed healthy fats, like salmon, sardines, walnuts, avocado, butter, coconut oil, and MCT oil.

Eating high-fat and low-carb allows the mitochondria to use those fatty acids or healthy carbohydrates to create the ATP. However, if you provide more fat and fewer carbs, fewer damaging free radicals are formed while allowing maintenance of the beneficial ones.

The kinds of carbs that will best nourish your mitochondria are colorful vegetables. Their numerous phytonutrients will nourish your mitochondria. Sulfur-rich veggies like cauliflower, cabbage, arugula, broccoli, Brussels sprouts, kale, radishes, watercress and bok choy produce glutathione, a powerful antioxidant that's good for the mitochondria.

Keep in mind if you choose to eat more healthy fats but still eat processed grain carbs, your cells will use the carbs first. This will result in having excess carbs or insulin and excess fat, which will cause weight gain. If you avoid the carbs, your body will process the fats. Mitochondria do better on fatty acids than carbohydrates, but they will go for the carbohydrates first if given the option.

Another way to strengthen your mitochondria is doing high intensity interval training (HIIT), as well as making sure to get adequate sleep and managing stress effectively. Certain supplements, like CoQ10, alpha lipoic acid, magnesium, D-ribose and fish oil are also nourishing to the mitochondria.

On to the microbiome.

At all times there are actually billions of beneficial bacteria present within all of us. These bacteria make up our microbiome, which is our inner ecosystem. That internal terrain is extraordinarily important for overall health. The microbiome is key for a strong immune system, keeping our digestive systems running smoothly, our hormone levels balanced and our brains working properly. The bulk of our microbiome lives in our gut, but the skin has its own, as do the eyes, the mouth, etc.

According to the Department of Chemistry & Biochemistry at the University of Colorado, "the human microbiota consists of the 10–100 trillion symbiotic microbial cells harbored by each person, primarily bacteria in the gut. The human 'microbiome' consists of the genes these cells harbor."

https://www.ncbi.nlm.nih.gov/pmc/articles/PMC3426293/

Your unique microbiome helps determine your unique DNA, hereditary factors, predisposition to diseases, body type, "set point weight," fertility and longevity. According to some experts 90% of all diseases can be traced in some way back to the gut and health of the microbiome. So I think you will agree keeping it healthy is of the utmost importance. So how do we do that?

In general, the foods you eat, how much you sleep, the amount of bacteria you're exposed to on a daily basis and the level of stress you live with all help establish the state of your microbiota. It is important to reduce inflammation and support the health of your digestive system in order to have a healthy, diverse microbiome.

Eliminating pro-inflammatory, refined vegetable oils and trans-fats, sugar, refined carbs and processed grains is an excellent start. Including lots of anti-inflammatory foods like vegetables of all kinds, including leafy greens, low sugar whole fruits (in moderation) like berries, apples and citrus, healthy fats like pasture butter, coconut oil, extra virgin olive and avocado oil, nuts, seeds, grass-fed and finished meats, which are high in anti-inflammatory Omega-3s, wild caught fish, cage free eggs, anti-inflammatory herbs and spices including turmeric, ginger, basil, oregano, thyme, cinnamon and cumin, and probiotics, as well as probiotic-rich foods like kefir, Amasai, yogurt, kombucha and cultured vegetables.

You will be able to see more clearly when we get to the specifics of this plan that it is full of these healthy foods that keep both your mitochondria and microbiome healthy.

Baby Steps: Small Changes = Big Impact

I've come to believe that the smaller changes make the biggest difference in most cases—especially when it comes to health.

According to research from a study published in the Journal of the American Geriatrics Society, for every 30 minute increase in moderate to vigorous physical activity in women aged 63 to 99, there was approximately a 40% reduction in all-cause mortality. Ok so that's no big surprise. Staying active and exercising definitely helps keep us strong and healthy.

What was surprising, however, is that the research also showed that 30 minutes of very light activity—like household chores or walking slowly over short distances—led to a 12% reduction in mortality.

This is important on several levels but particularly because when people think that only big changes can make a difference, they aren't likely to take action. If someone who is completely sedentary thinks she has to hit the gym for an hour five days a week to improve her health, she might be so overwhelmed that she ends up doing nothing at all.

But what if he or she knows that even light activity, such as gardening, taking the stairs instead of the elevator, or walking a half-mile to the store instead of driving can make a meaningful difference? Chances are they will be a lot more likely to do it.

Once you simply add a little more activity and movement to your day, you'll feel better, more confident, and more empowered to take the next step. One positive baby step leads to another and creates powerful, positive momentum. I told you baby steps are powerful!

The same is true with making changes to your eating plan. Deciding to give up sweets, bread, pasta and soda cold turkey and all at once is a recipe (pardon the pun) for disaster! It is much more effective to make one of those changes gradually and stick with that for several weeks until it becomes your new natural, and then make a second change. That is the beauty of baby steps.

It's not a race or a competition. The only person you are trying to be better than is the you from yesterday! You don't have to do it all at once. Actually, that almost never works. Commit to taking baby steps and you will be surprised at the difference they make.

Consistency and Variety

While baby steps are definitely the way to go, there is another aspect we need to touch on and that is consistency. What good is replacing one soda with a glass of water for four days and then going right back to the old habits?

In order to make continued, steady progress toward your goals using baby steps, you must be consistent. Turning that consistency into a habit takes some time. Most people say 21 days, but brain researcher, Dr. Caroline Leaf has studied this and finds that it takes 21 days to rewire neural pathways in the brain and begin building a new thought pattern. It then takes another 42 days (for a total of 63) to establish that new habit or thought! I think the first point is that we have to be a little more patient and a lot more consistent and intentional about making these changes so they are long-term and not just temporary changes.

Before you throw your hands up and decide it's too difficult, think about this. You have been successful at being consistent all your life. You automatically brush your teeth and comb your hair in the morning. You don't have to think about it or make a new decision every day. You just do it. That is what you want to create with these new habits you are going to develop as we move through the program.

The longer and more consistently you practice them, the easier they will become and you will find they are your new natural.

While it is very important, particularly at the beginning, to be consistent and not deviate from the plan, once it has become your new normal, you will be able to stray from the plan occasionally without it setting you back to the beginning. Holidays come around each year and if you are honest, you will eat your favorite foods and enjoy them. And there's nothing wrong with that! In fact, I think it is healthy and helpful to vary your meals periodically. It keeps your body surprised, just as varying your workout routine does.

The point is to make it a few days (not a few weeks) and to go back to your new normal as quickly as possible.

Pick Your Poison: Factors That Could be Stalling Weight Loss

I'm sure I don't have to convince you that stress is harmful to your health.

"Stress is a factor in five out of the six leading causes of death — heart disease, cancer, stroke, lower respiratory disease, and accidents. An estimated 75 percent to 90 percent of all doctor visits are for stress-related issues. ... The culprit behind so many of our health problems is staring us in the face." Huffington Post

Ok, so we are in agreement that stress causes health problems. A recent study indicates that too much stress may be as destructive to health as junk food. So when I say pick your poison, I am referring to stress and junk food!

What I found especially fascinating about the study was that stress and a junk food diet had different effects on males and females. Male mice on the high-fat diet* showed more anxiety than females on the high-fat diet, and high-fat males also showed decreased activity in response to stress. However, it was only in female mice that stress caused the microbiome composition in the gut to shift as if they were on a high-fat diet. Stress changed the bacteria to resemble that of obese mice!

*Keep in mind when they say a high-fat diet it is not referring to healthy fats, but to the kind in processed, fast and junk foods.

So many women I happen to know and some I work with are under so much stress on a daily basis that they find it becomes almost impossible to lose weight. They become frustrated and discouraged, and that adds more stress – a vicious cycle. Even when they clean up their diet and begin eating well, some still find it very difficult to lose weight and begin blaming themselves when it could all come down to too much stress.

If that sounds too simplistic, consider this: Due to the hormonal changes it creates, stress causes cravings and continual feelings of hunger, making it much more difficult to lose weight; it raises blood sugar and causes the accumulation of belly fat, the most hormonally active and dangerous kind; high stress makes it almost impossible for your body to break down fat, so you end up storing more; stress is linked to mood disorders like depression, anxiety and unhappiness which can be triggers for overeating; and stress hinders the ability to sleep, raising cortisol levels, which is also linked to weight gain.

Obviously this study was done with mice, but the researchers felt confident it could have important impacts for us as well.

While we are on this subject, let me touch briefly on just a few other reasons you may find your weight loss efforts stalled.

Consuming too much fructose. Most sugars trigger a rise in blood sugar and insulin levels, whereas fructose is directly metabolized in the liver. When you get too much fructose, that excess is converted into fat! This is why I recommend limiting fruit to two servings, and if you eliminate sodas and other sugary foods and beverages, you will reduce fructose intake.

I must mention snacking here. Every time you eat, you raise your insulin levels. When insulin levels are elevated, fat-burning is shut down. To tap into your fat stores and burn what you've already got stored requires taking a break between meals. Snacking between meals interrupts that process. This is why intermittent fasting has become such a popular way to structure meals. I will talk more about this in the chapter on fasting coming up.

Besides stimulating your appetite and interrupting sound sleep, drinking alcohol will shut down fat burning because your body prioritizes metabolizing alcohol first. According to research, alcohol intake is one of the leading (and perhaps overlooked) causes of high cholesterol and triglyceride levels as well.

I recommend not eating past 7 pm in this plan, and research confirms that eating late at night can increase your weight and impair fat metabolism, putting you at a greater risk of obesity and the health issues that go along with it.

There is an entire chapter devoted to the importance of sleep and rest and for good reason: going without sleep knocks your stress- and appetite-regulating hormones out of whack, making you feel hungrier and more likely to succumb to emotional eating. It is a stressor in and of itself. Inadequate sleep causes a rise in insulin levels which triggers fat storage.

My take-away is this: Yes, it is important to eat a clean, whole food diet, but it is just as critical to be aware of other factors, like stress and lack of sleep, which we all experience to one degree or another, and to acknowledge how they could be affecting your efforts at weight loss and health.

Better than BMI: Waist Management

You may have been told to track your BMI, Body Mass Index, in order to determine whether you are overweight or obese. I offered ways to calculate your BMI in the original Today's the Day plan and have since changed my thoughts on using this as a tool.

BMI has drawn criticism as to whether it's an accurate assessment of health since a high BMI does not take into account muscle mass and other critical factors that may impact health. BMI indirectly measures body composition calculating it on height and weight without measuring fat. So if you have a great deal of muscle mass, your BMI could categorize you as obese when you truly are not. If you have a high amount of body fat but are normal or low weight, it may show your BMI as normal when that may not be the case.

Research suggests that even if your weight is in the normal range, if you have a high waist-to-hip ratio, you have a higher risk of death than those considered obese based on BMI. Waist size has been shown to be a more effective indication of visceral (deep) fat levels which have been linked to the development of Type 2 diabetes, cardiovascular disease and certain cancers. Your waist size is a powerful indicator of insulin sensitivity.

Although everyone should know their own waist measurement, those who have a BMI within the normal range may find the most benefit from tracking this measurement. Some people who have a normal BMI may carry much of their weight in their stomach, which increases their risk for chronic diseases. For men, waist-circumference levels should be below 40 inches, and for women it should be below 35 inches.

An even more accurate way to use this measurement is to calculate your waist-to-hip ratio (WHR). It is simple to do. Measure your waist at the smallest circumference of your natural waist, just above your belly button. Measure the circumference of your hips at the widest part, across your buttocks. Then divide your waist measurement by your hip measurement to get the ratio.

In both men and women, a WHR of 1.0 or higher increases the risk for heart disease and other conditions that are linked to being overweight. For women, a WHR of 0.80 or lower is indicative of low health risk, and for men, WHR should be 0.95 or lower.

People shorter than five feet tall and those with a BMI of 35 or higher won't be able to get an accurate measure using WHR, but for most people, it's a simple and accurate way to track fat loss.

Non-Scale Ways to Track Progress

While weighing once a week is a valid way to track your progress, many women have a love-hate relationship with the scale. When the numbers on the scale go down, they feel they are making progress. If they don't budge for a week or two or even go up a pound, they panic. Some people weigh daily and start stressing if they fluctuate by more than a pound. That's counter-productive. If you weigh, once a week is more than enough.

But that's not the only way to measure how well your efforts are succeeding. It doesn't always tell the whole story either, so besides waist circumference and measuring waist-to-hip ratio, here are a few other ways to track your progress without using the scale.

Pay attention to how your clothes fit. Looser pants equal progress. When you lose fat, which is the goal, your body composition changes. The number on the scale may stay the same or even go up a pound or two, but if your pants are loose, it is indicative of fat loss. This is why you also track your measurements and not just your weight.

A picture is worth a thousand words. Take a picture of yourself when you begin and do so intermittently. Look at the photos and compare them. When you see yourself daily, often you don't see the subtle changes taking place. But you can see the difference in pictures.

How do you feel? Can you climb a flight of stairs without getting out of breath? Are you able to exercise longer? Do you feel less exhausted at the end of the day? Do you notice less joint pain?

All of those are indicators of progress.

If you had blood work done when you began, you will most likely see significant improvements the next time you visit the doctor. Your blood pressure may go down, cholesterol and blood sugar levels will normalize. These are excellent markers of progress that you should celebrate.

So, the scale is not the only indicator of progress. It may not even be the best.

Fasting

You may be hearing and reading about intermittent fasting and wondering what it is and whether you should consider it. Intermittent fasting describes an eating pattern that cycles between periods of fasting and eating, feasting and famine.

While there are numerous potential health benefits from fasting, including improved immune function, increased growth hormone, more energy, and fat loss, it's not for everyone. If you have adrenal fatigue, gallbladder disease or gallstones, issues with stress, fertility, thyroid or blood sugar balance, it may not be your best choice. Women tend to be more sensitive to skipping meals than men, so it's important to pay attention to how any change affects you personally. For women, fasting could lead to hormonal imbalance and fertility issues if done incorrectly. However, there are some ways women can enjoy the positive aspects of intermittent fasting without putting their health at risk. This research article details the benefits of fasting specific to women.

https://www.ncbi.nlm.nih.gov/pmc/articles/PMC4960941/

According to Dr. Amy Shah, women are extremely sensitive to signals of starvation, and if the body senses that it is being starved, it will ramp up production of the hunger hormones leptin and ghrelin, making fasting extremely difficult. Her recommendation is to practice what she calls "crescendo fasting." Here's how she recommends doing it:

Ideally, fast for 12–16 hours on two to three nonconsecutive days per week (ex. Tuesday, Thursday, Saturday).

On fasting days, do light cardio.

Eat normally on your strength training/HIIT workout days.

Drink plenty of water. (Tea and coffee are okay, too, as long as there is no added milk or sweetener.)

After two weeks, feel free to add one more day of fasting if you want to.

Another easy way to reap many of the health benefits without the drawbacks is to give yourself a 12- to 16-hour overnight fast. This is how I practice intermittent fasting. This is very easy to do if you do not eat past 7 pm and then wait an hour or two to have breakfast. This way you are doing the bulk of your fasting during the night while you sleep and then if you limit your meals to an eight hour window – say between 10 am and 6 pm you -- will be reaping the most benefits. You can do this several times a week – it doesn't have to be every day.

Studies show by simply restricting eating to an 8-10 hour window, daily caloric intake was reduced by up to 20%!

Fasting is one of the oldest dietary interventions known to man. It's literally been around forever. Fasting is an extremely powerful way to influence health and besides intermittent fasting as described above, there are other variations you may consider:

Water fasting. This is exactly what it sounds like: You don't eat; you only drink water, for several days in a row (typically no less than 24 hours).

Water plus non-caloric beverages. A slight variation on the water fast is to include other non-caloric beverages, such as herbal tea and coffee (without milk, sugar or other sweetener, including artificial non-caloric sweeteners).

Bone broth fast. Another variation for longer fasts is using bone broth. In addition to healthy fats, bone broth also contains lots of protein, so it's not really a true fast but effective nonetheless. Just drinking quality bone broth instead of meals for 24 hours is an easy and effective way to reset yourself after a day or two of not eating right and provides so many extra benefits. It's one of my favorite ways to fast, especially during cold winter months.

Fat fasting. In this variation, healthy fats are included during the fast in addition to water and/or non-caloric beverages. You could have bulletproof coffee or tea (black coffee or tea with butter, coconut oil or MCT oil).

Fasting is safe for most people; however, if you are underweight, malnourished, a child, pregnant or breastfeeding, you should not fast. Also, if you are on any type of pharmaceutical medication, you need to exercise caution and check with your doctor before making any dietary changes.

Fasting allows your digestive tract to "rest and digest!" By giving your digestion a break, you help heal damage to your gut lining, like leaky gut, which may be causing you to have low immunity and/or inflammation.

Is There One "Best" Diet?

I know and work with people who ascribe to all different diets for various reasons. I don't particularly like to use labels because I think diet should be fluid and change as the needs in life arise. A gentleman asked me if I was a WFPB eater. I had no idea what that was, so I looked it up and I think it comes closest to describing how I eat most of the time – whole food, plant based, but with quality animal protein.

In the past I've even called myself a "qualitarian" – the quality of the food, whether animal foods or produce, is what matters most to me. A vegetarian who eats genetically modified fruits and vegetables and lots of grains is definitely *not* going to be healthier than someone who chooses grass-fed, pasture-raised and wild-caught animal foods along with organic produce. It's not quite as cut and dried as some would have you believe. That's why I say:

Eating meat as opposed to a totally vegetarian or vegan diet doesn't matter as much as the quality of the food.

Dr. Mark Hyman, author of *"Eat Fat, Get Thin"* says:

"It's not easy to know for sure what the truth is. Vegan diet studies show they help with weight loss, reverse diabetes, and lower cholesterol. Diets high in fat and animal protein seem to do the same thing. Essentially, each scientist (or even each person reading the research) with a point of view adheres to his or her position with near religious fervor. Each can point to studies validating his or her perspective."

I think Dr. Hyman hit the nail on the head and I totally agree. Besides the fact that quality of food is of the utmost importance, each person's metabolism and biochemistry is different. Their system can change over time and during specific seasons in life. What worked well in your 20s may not be so good for you at 45. That was certainly my experience and how I came to develop this plan.

While studies show vegan diets help with weight loss, it is not true for me. This is why I do not think anyone can say with 100% certainty that any one particular diet is "best" for everyone. This study bears that out. Regardless of what diet you choose or prefer, the ultimate goal is to live a longer, healthier life. This study concluded "there was no significant difference in all-cause mortality for vegetarians versus non-vegetarians."

https://www.ncbi.nlm.nih.gov/pubmed/28040519

So why don't we stop trying to convince each other our way is best and each just make the best choices available for ourselves. It's not a contest after all – we all seem to want the same thing: *to live a long, healthy, active life. It makes no difference if we approach it in slightly different ways as long as the result is the same.*

It's All About Results

Before we get into the nitty-gritty of the plan, I have two questions for you.

What will it take for you to commit to making these changes? Are you really ready to take action?

It doesn't matter how good this all sounds to you if you are not moved to take action. It's all about results. If you read this book from cover to cover but never implement any of the recommendations, you will have increased your knowledge but it does nothing to help you live a healthier life.

Kenneth Copeland calls it making a "quality decision." I have learned from experience working with many different people that each of us must have a specific, personal reason that moves us to action.

For one client, it was a diagnosis of pre-diabetes. For another, it was in preparation for starting her family. For someone else, it was to set a better example for her husband and family. For another, it was to relieve knee pain and be able to walk freely. It is unique to each of us. It is critical that you find what matters to you the most.

It is not enough to stick to a diet plan for a certain number of weeks and then go right back to your old way of eating and think you can maintain the results. In all honesty, releasing weight is not the most challenging part of this. Often it is the easiest part. The challenge comes with maintaining the change long-term.

If you just want to get to a certain number on the scale for a wedding or reunion, then any "diet" will probably work for you. If, however, your goal is not only to get to a healthier weight, but to improve your overall health, then whether you realize it or not, what you are seeking to do is change your lifestyle in a way that you can sustain for the long-haul.

While the thought of that may seem overwhelming, remember one of the basic principles of this plan is taking baby steps. You can always move at your own pace. You never have to change everything all at once to experience improvement.

So before you turn the page, honestly and carefully think about *why* you want to do this. Keep that reason front and center before you as you move ahead. You can jump ahead to the end of Week Seven: Putting It All Together, Integrating Spirit and Soul Practices and see the suggestions for crafting a compelling "why" in the soul section.

Remember - no action, no results.

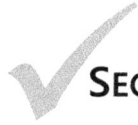

✓ SECTION TWO

THE BASIC TODAY IS STILL THE DAY PLAN

Introduction

"What has been will be again, what has been done will be done again; there is nothing new under the sun." (Ecclesiastes 1:9) It's very true, particularly of weight loss and fitness plans. There are hundreds of "diets" out there. It can be pretty overwhelming trying to choose a plan that's right for you.

You are a unique one-of-a-kind creation—one size doesn't fit all—especially when it comes to health and nutrition. We are all bio-chemically unique. I have found the most effective approach is to put basic, foundational principles for good health in place and then customize them for your particular needs and physiology. This fitness plan incorporates wisdom and principles from the Bible as well as from respected health and fitness experts.

Many of the diets advertised on TV focus on being able to eat pizza, cake and ice cream and still lose weight. Of course you have to buy their pizza, cake and ice cream. That's very short-sighted in my opinion, because it doesn't help you make long-term changes unless you intend to buy the prepared foods forever, and it ignores overall health and just focuses on weight loss. Quick fixes don't work because they don't involve changing habits. They don't involve making sustainable changes. They unfortunately often involve unhealthy, short-term tactics.

Maintaining a healthy weight is a critical factor in overall health. "Diets," particularly restrictive diets, are not a healthy alternative and they have a very high failure rate. If you cannot sustain the "diet" and make it part of your everyday life, you will abandon it and go right back to the eating habits that created your excess weight in the first place.

Another factor many "diets" don't address is the quality of the fuel you put in your body. One lady I worked with told me she had great success with a well-known diet plan in the past, but that it was no longer working for her no matter how hard she tried. She counted points faithfully and stuck to the program with no success. Then she described a typical day's meals—which included eating frozen whipped topping as an approved snack! Frozen whipped topping contains chemicals and trans-fats and cannot by any stretch of the imagination be considered "food," much less healthy fuel!

This plan is based on my 3-D Living Program, which is based on fresh, whole, nutrient-dense foods. When you eat real food that provides your body with the vitamins, minerals, fiber, enzymes, fats and co-factors it needs in order to perform the functions that keep it working at peak performance, you naturally eat less, have more energy, and maintain a healthy weight easily.

The number of calories consumed is, of course, important in losing and maintaining a healthy weight, but what many diets fail to consider is the quality of those calories as I mentioned in an earlier chapter. The fuel needs to be real food! Unless you provide real, nutrient-dense whole food your body recognizes as food, you simply fill your belly and satisfy the momentary hunger. Without providing nutrients your body needs at the cellular level to maintain health, you simply fill your belly (and expand your waistline) while starving yourself at the cellular level. You can be overweight or even obese and malnourished at the same time, and many people are!

I have called it "*Today is Still the Day*" based on Exodus 8:9-10: when Moses told Pharaoh to decide when he should rid the land of the frogs. Unbelievably, Pharaoh said, "Tomorrow!!" How often do we do the same thing? I'll start a diet tomorrow—begin exercising tomorrow—stop drinking diet soda tomorrow. There is no "tomorrow!" There is only today. So Today's the Day! Today is STILL the Day! Don't wait a minute longer! If you are wondering why seven weeks, seven is the number of perfection in the Bible, and science has proven our body regenerates cells and tissues, creating a new body approximately every seven years.

This plan is based on my 3-D Living Plan, which applies four simple keys: Detox, Fuel, Exercise, and Rest to spirit, soul and body.

The primary reason for the failure of most diets is that you can't make it a lifestyle. This system is the way I eat every day. You can adapt this to fit your lifestyle in any way you need to and, in fact, this is what I do with clients in the companion coaching. The biggest change is in how you think: about food, eating, your body and being healthy overall. I deal with spiritual issues as well as mental and emotional (soul) issues that will sabotage your efforts if left unaddressed.

This is why I call it living a 3D life of wholeness. It is what sets this plan apart from 99% of the popular plans. You cannot just address your eating and physical habits and overlook your thoughts, emotions and beliefs.

All that is required of you is to make the commitment to seven weeks and give it 100% effort. If a question arises as you move through the plan, you can always email me and I will clarify anything you are stuck on.

Overview Of The Plan

For those who like to get the Big Picture and know exactly what it will look like going forward, here's the plan in a nutshell:

Pre-Plan Preparation – Clean out your kitchen and pantry.

Order any supplements you choose to use and get plan-friendly foods in the house.

Begin a simple food and exercise log to track daily progress.

Begin gradually increasing your water intake to get to one-half your body weight in ounces with ¼ teaspoon of natural, unprocessed salt for every 32 ounces of water.

Fill out your Personal Commitment Contract.

Weeks 1 and 2: Detox Weeks. Create your meals around clean protein, non-starchy vegetables and healthy fats. No starchy carbs or grains at all in these two weeks. Also pay attention to Spirit/Soul detox in Section Three.

Weeks 3 and 4: Nourish and Fuel. You can now include one small serving of a healthy, friendly carb (starchy vegetable or grain) at either breakfast *or* lunch (not both) *if* you choose to. You can also remain on the detox part of the plan for the duration of the plan, or just add in the healthy carbs on the weekends. See what works for you. Also pay attention to nourishing and fueling your spirit and soul, in Section Three.

Week 5: Intentional Activity/Exercise. If you haven't already, here is where you can begin to include some intentional activity in your day. Walking is one of the easiest and safest forms of exercise available to just about everyone. Pay attention to exercising your spirit, mind, will and emotions as well (see Section Three).

Week 6: Rest and Reboot. Here is where you address your sleep habits, as they will impact your ability to successfully release weight. Reboot refers to rest and relaxation. You need to carve out a few minutes throughout the day to just disconnect and rest – physically. Also, you will learn ways to rest and reboot spiritually, mentally and emotionally as well in Section Three.

Week 7: Putting it All Together. Here is where I give you some ideas of how incorporating these principles into your daily life can look going forward. If you can't make it part of your life, then it's just a temporary change, and that's not what we are after here. There is a corresponding chapter in Section Three for integrating the spirit and soul principles.

Ok, now let's get down to the nitty-gritty!

Pre-Plan Preparation

Clean out the kitchen and pantry. Get rid of white flour products like cookies, cakes, pastas and white bread, candies, sodas (high sugar and high fructose corn syrup products), processed, packaged foods, and hydrogenated (bad) fats and refined oils, margarine, artificial sweeteners, and processed, white table salt.

Ok, maybe you're thinking—so now my kitchen is bare! What's left? Plenty! Here is a suggested list of foods to stock up on:

Shopping List

High Quality Protein

Pasture raised poultry—chicken, turkey, Cornish hen;

Wild caught fish— salmon, tuna, sardines, mackerel, herring, flounder, sole, cod;

Ground chicken, turkey, bison, lean grass-fed beef, veal or lamb;

Chicken Sausage (Al Fresco and Aidells are two good brands);

Natural Choice or Applegate Naturals cold cuts (no nitrates or nitrites) *occasionally*;

Eggs—Omega-3 or cage free, organic, if possible;

Whey, collagen, hemp, pea, cranberry or rice protein powder.

Starting your day with a complete, clean protein is extremely important on many levels. Complete proteins like clean, grass-fed animal meats, eggs or a quality protein shake will increase chemicals in the brain that not only improve sleep but also improve your mood due to their tryptophan content. This amino acid is a precursor to serotonin. Serotonin is our "feel-good hormone" and makes us feel happy and motivated throughout the day. Serotonin then turns into melatonin, which helps us sleep at night! Fewer than six hours of sleep per day is associated with low-grade chronic inflammation and worsening insulin resistance, as well as increased risk for obesity, Type 2 diabetes, and cardiovascular disease. Without that complete protein at the start of the day, this conversion can't take place, leaving you tired, moody and possibly overweight!

A recent study suggests that adequate protein in the morning helps tame appetite throughout the day.

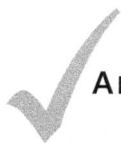

ANN'S PERSONAL TIP

It is especially important to include clean protein with breakfast. Studies prove that starting the day with a form of clean protein instead of carbs can reduce risk of fatigue by up to 75% for six hours and double your energy within 30 minutes. One study found women who included protein in their breakfast meal lost weight 65% faster!

Non-Starchy Vegetables: Choose organic whenever possible.

Fresh or frozen chopped spinach (this is a great, fast addition to omelets, smoothies and burgers); Romaine, red and green leaf or whatever lettuces you love; artichokes, parsley, cilantro, beets, kale, tomato, broccoli, cabbage, cauliflower, cucumbers, Brussels sprouts, eggplant, bell peppers, Swiss chard, mushrooms, squash (zucchini, yellow summer), celery, sprouts (alfalfa, broccoli), arugula, radicchio, broccoli rabe, broccolini, collard greens, escarole, endive, onions, green beans, radishes, garlic, watercress, asparagus; low sodium V-8 Juice (If you have joint issues, avoid nightshades like tomatoes, bell peppers and eggplant).

Healthy Fats: Extra virgin olive oil, virgin coconut oil*, avocado oil, flax seed oil, hemp oil, MCT oil, pasture butter, organic ghee; olives, avocados;

unsalted, organic, raw nuts and seeds like almonds, chestnuts, macadamias, walnuts, cashews, pine nuts, pistachios, sesame, chia, flax, hemp, pumpkin and sunflower seeds.

*Coconut oil is one of the best fats you can use for so many reasons. It has been shown to increase metabolism by up to 48% in normal weight people and up to 65% in obese people, and that increase lasts for 24 hours. A great food for your weight loss arsenal!

Fresh or frozen organic fruits: apples (especially Granny Smith), bananas, avocado, mangoes, oranges, lemons, grapefruit, cherries, strawberries, blueberries, raspberries, blackberries, pineapple, pears, peaches.

Beans and legumes: lentils, peas, black, red kidney, pink, garbanzo, cannellini, Adzuki beans - ¼ to 1/2 cup a day after the first two detox weeks. While beans and legumes are not the only sources of lectins, they are a primary source. Frequent consumption of large amounts of lectins can damage the intestinal lining. Pressure cooking beans or purchasing the Eden brand, which are pressure cooked, eliminates this problem as it destroys the lectins.

Natural, Unprocessed salt: Celtic Sea Salt, Himalayan Crystal Salt or Pink Salt; Herbamare (available in most health food stores), which has a combination of sea salt and 12 organic herbs and vegetables.

Herbs and spices: whichever you love, but try and include black pepper (which is shown to make fat cells less likely to develop, grow or multiply), cinnamon, (which helps stabilize blood sugar and lowers inflammation), ginger, garlic, cayenne pepper, fennel, dill, turmeric, coriander and cumin. They all accelerate metabolism, aid digestion and improve insulin and glucose levels.

You may include Nutritional Yeast Seasoning – I buy Bragg's from my health food store, which is loaded with B vitamins, protein and is gluten free; Maine Coast Sea Seasonings Organic Dulse Granules, Bragg's Organic Sea Kelp Delight Seasoning or Eden Seaweed Gomasio, which are good sources of iodine – all healthy, tasty seasonings that boost nutrition and thyroid health.

Apple Cider Vinegar: raw, organic and unfiltered (Bragg's is a good brand; balsamic vinegar is good, too); fresh lemons, organic where possible. I also like Coconut Aminos as a replacement for soy sauce.

Teas: including Tulsi, yerba mate, hibiscus, black, white, matcha, Rooibos, green, or oolong tea daily and any herbal tea you really like. Ginger and peppermint are great for digestion. You can add a squeeze of lemon to green tea to get more of the nutritional value. My morning tea includes a tablespoon of pasture butter, a tablespoon of MCT oil and a scoop of collagen powder. I usually combine two or more different teas – I believe in getting the most bang for my nutritional buck.

If you are a coffee drinker, that's ok in moderation and as long as it is a clean, high quality coffee.

Sweeteners: stevia, Lakanto or erythritol, raw, organic honey or organic maple syrup, in moderation.

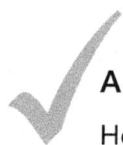

ANN'S PERSONAL TIP

Here's an extra strategy you may want to include: try eating off a salad plate which is smaller than a regular dinner plate, or use a plate that has a wide border around the edge. Also use a large fork as opposed to a dessert fork. Both will help you reduce the amount of food you serve yourself, helping with portion control.

We'll talk more about how to make some tasty meals that will satisfy your taste buds and appetite, help your body release toxins and fuel your metabolism.

Order Supplements:

You can do the Plan without using any supplements. However, sometimes we feel the need for a little extra help. The ones I recommend are all natural, so you might want to consider adding at least one or two to your arsenal. *Please note that any marked with an asterisk are ones I sell. If you purchase them, I receive a commission.

Visit the resource page here: http://www.threedimensionalvitality.com/resource-page-for-book.html or https://bit.ly/2Eqo1sb. You will find a list of supplements I use and recommend and links to purchase, should you decide to. I am putting this information separately because links change often and I can keep that list up to date for you. Of course you can also purchase from a local health food store as well. If you choose to use them, I suggest ordering or purchasing during the pre-plan, get ready period so you have them on hand when you begin.

Here are a few of the basic supplements you might consider including:

Multi vitamin mineral supplement. This is something I think we all need since our food supply is compromised and no one eats perfectly. It's just smart to cover your nutritional bases. I suggest Beyond Tangy Tangerine 2.0. I use the powder, but it comes in pill form as well.

CLA. Research indicates CLA (conjugated lineoleic acid) increases fat loss and prevents fat regain by helping maintain lean body mass; it enhances fat metabolism naturally, safely and without stimulants.

Omega-3 supplement. Cod liver, salmon or krill oil; essential for overall health, cardiovascular health, reduced inflammation.

Fiber supplement. It is essential to keep yourself regular, especially when detoxing. Fiber can be added in several different ways. Most people do not get enough fiber and it is important not only in keeping you regular, but also in stabilizing blood sugar, removing toxins and escorting fat from the body, making your body work harder to digest your meal when taken before eating. Fiber lowers the glycemic index of meals and it expands to many times its volume making you feel fuller more quickly.

You can use konjac root (Glucomannan) fiber capsules before meals or use ground flax seeds or psyllium fiber powder in smoothies. If you use flax seeds, be sure to buy them ground or grind them before using if purchasing whole seeds. If you don't, they'll just pass through your system and you will not get the benefit they provide.

Also, using aloe juice daily during the detox weeks is another option that will keep your system functioning and soothe your digestive system.

Digestive Enzyme and Probiotic. Helping your body to effectively digest your meals helps prevent food from sitting (and fermenting and putrefying!) in your digestive tract causing more toxins. Probiotics enhance immune function and digestion as well.

There are some other helpful supplements you might want to consider now or in the future, and you'll find the information and links for them on the resource page.

Prepare your food and exercise log:

Get a notebook—any kind will do—to keep track of your daily progress—this is very important. List every food and drink you consume with specific amounts and how you feel after the meal. I have provided a sample meal log page at the end of this chapter.

**Don't ignore this step! A recent study suggests that weight loss is increased by six pounds simply by keeping a food log.

On page one of your notebook, note the date you begin the plan as well as these stats: (There's a sample log page for your stats you can print out at the end of this chapter)

- ✓ *Weight*
- ✓ *Note your goal for these seven weeks such as:*
- ✓ *Measurements**
- ✓ *Release __ pounds;*
- ✓ *Be able to walk five miles easily;*
- ✓ *Lose one or two clothing sizes.*

Be realistic!

**I use the term "release" rather than "lose" because your mind is very sensitive to the words you speak and if you lose something, chances are you will find it again and that's not what you want. It may seem silly and picky but trust me, little things like this make a difference.

*If you are wondering exactly how to take your measurements—here's how:

Using a flexible tape measure, flex your bicep and measure the biggest part, and that's your arm measurement; using a mirror, look to the side and measure the biggest part of your butt, and this is your hip measurement; measure around your belly, even with your belly button; measure the narrowest part of your waist and for your chest, measure just above the nipple, with your breath out; measure around the top of your thigh. Measure again at the end of the seven weeks.

I suggest you weigh once a week, preferably on the same day and approximately at the same time each week—and note it in your log. It will be exciting when you begin seeing the number on the scale decrease and feel your clothes get looser!

Increase Hydration:

The goal is to be drinking one-half your body weight in ounces daily and using ¼ teaspoon of unprocessed sea salt, Himalayan crystal salt or Pink salt per 32 ounces daily. Begin to increase water intake gradually - adding 8-16 ounces per day until you reach the amount you need to be drinking daily. This is very important - proper hydration makes a huge difference in whether you will release weight or not, and I factor it into your daily meal plans. **If you do not drink adequate water in order to see your weight drop as some who use drastic weight loss methods do—you risk dehydration and serious health issues. Also, you will not be losing FAT, which is the goal, but simply losing water and damaging muscle and tissue in the process. This is of critical importance. **

Natural, unprocessed salt prevents dehydration. If your body lacks salt, it cannot hold water. Salt is the essential compound that allows your body to hold and move water throughout your body's 100 trillion cells. Without salt, any person or animal will die of dehydration. See the chapter, "Water and Salt – Why?" in Section One for more information on the importance of salt.

Personal Commitment Contract:

See the "Today is Still the Day" Commitment Contract on the next page. I suggest you print it out—fill it out and sign it and post it where you will be sure to see it EVERY DAY! Keeping your goal front and center in your mind and before your eyes is a powerful incentive, especially on those days when you feel like quitting – and we all have them.

Extras:

While we will go into detail about exercise in week five, feel free to begin walking for at least 30 minutes daily. If you haven't exercised in a long time—check with your doctor—and with his ok, begin slowly - 10 minutes a day and work up to at least 30 minutes for five days a week.

If you use this time to prepare yourself and your kitchen, you'll find it so much easier to slip into this new, healthier routine!

Are you getting excited?? You should be—this is going to be amazing!

TODAY IS STILL THE DAY!

PERSONAL COMMITMENT CONTRACT

I, _____ do hereby commit to the following goals within the next 7 weeks:

_____

_____

_____

- ✓ I am committed to achieving my fitness goals.
- ✓ I believe I am worth this effort and I know that success is inevitable.
- ✓ I have the support in place that I need in order to achieve my goals.
- ✓ I promise to make myself a priority.
- ✓ I will schedule time to take care of myself by following the plan and maintaining
  a positive attitude.
- ✓ I will speak faith confessions daily, building my spirit and faith.
- ✓ I will take action every day towards my goals and will never give up no matter what obstacles arise.

Feel free to add any others that particularly speak to you:

_____

_____

_____

"I can do all things, including reaching my goal, through Christ Who strengthens & empowers me!" *Philippians 4:13*

Signed: _____

Dated: _____

LOG STATS PAGE

My health goals are:

Examples:

- ✓ TO RELEASE 10 POUNDS IN THESE SEVEN WEEKS.
- ✓ TO DROP ONE DRESS SIZE.
- ✓ TO EAT A BALANCED BREAKFAST EVERY DAY.
- ✓ TO EXERCISE MOST DAYS OF THE WEEK.

MY PRIMARY GOAL IS:

Release 10 pounds of fat in these seven weeks and incorporate new eating habits.

Declaration: I WILL RELEASE 10 POUNDS IN THESE SEVEN WEEKS.

- ✓ PRESENT WEIGHT: _____
- ✓ WEIGHT AT END OF WEEK ONE: _____
- ✓ WEIGHT AT END OF WEEK TWO: _____
- ✓ WEIGHT AT END OF WEEK THREE: _____
- ✓ WEIGHT AT END OF WEEK FOUR: _____
- ✓ WEIGHT AT END OF WEEK FIVE: _____
- ✓ WEIGHT AT END OF WEEK SIX: _____
- ✓ WEIGHT AT END OF WEEK SEVEN: _____

MEASUREMENTS AT START:	MEASUREMENTS AFTER SEVEN WEEKS:
BICEP/ARM:	BICEP/ARM:
WAIST:	WAIST:
HIPS:	HIPS:
BELLY:	BELLY:
CHEST:	CHEST:
THIGH: L/R:	THIGH: L/R:
Waist/Hip Ratio:	Waist/Hip Ratio:

Water/salt requirement: _____ ounces of water and _____ teaspoon salt daily.

MEAL LOG PAGE

Simply note everything as accurately as possible:

DATE: _____

BREAKFAST – APPROXIMATE TIME OF MEAL: _____

FOODS:

BEVERAGES:

COMMENTS:

LUNCH – APPROXIMATE TIME OF MEAL: _____

FOODS:

BEVERAGES:

COMMENTS:

DINNER – APPROXIMATE TIME OF MEAL: _____

FOODS:

BEVERAGES:

SNACKS: TIME EATEN: _____; _____

FOOD:

BEVERAGES:

COMMENTS:

PLEASE NOTE IN THE COMMENTS – DID THE FOOD(S) CAUSE ANY DIGESTIVE DISTURBANCE? BLOATING? PAIN? CONSTIPATION? DIARRHEA? HAVE INDIGESTION?

WERE YOU HUNGRY SOON AFTER? JITTERY? LIGHT-HEADED? BRAIN FOG? RASHES?

NOTE HOW YOU SLEPT THAT NIGHT AFTER YOUR LAST MEAL OR SNACK.

WEEKS ONE AND TWO
BODY DETOX

So maybe you are wondering why begin with detox? The short answer is: simply because we live in such a toxic world. Not only is the air, water and food supply full of toxic substances, but there are toxic emotions, beliefs, thoughts and relationships that affect your overall health and well-being.

Detoxing your spirit and soul begins with honesty. Are there areas where you are resentful, bitter, holding onto a grudge or offense, unwilling to forgive, living with regret, guilt or shame? These are serious spiritual toxins that will affect your health as surely as ingesting poison would.

Your soul (mind, will and emotions) also must be kept clean and clear of toxic debris. Do you have constant negative thoughts running through your mind like an endless tape? Are you constantly dealing with emotions like fear, anxiety or anger? Do you feel unable to make healthier choices and stick with them? Again, these are toxins. We will get into this in more detail in Section Three: Spirit and Soul Detox. Right now we will focus on the body.

Physically, some of the symptoms of a toxic body include: increased inflammation (the root of most disease); hormonal imbalances; insulin resistance; increased stress response; reduced thyroid hormone levels; compromised metabolism, which hinders your ability to release and maintain a healthy weight; congested, overloaded liver and kidneys - your main organs of detoxification.

A congested, toxic liver hinders your ability to burn calories efficiently and to release weight. Clean, quality protein, like whey, is important because protein unclogs the liver and activates fat burning. Whey protein in particular contains special peptides that increase glutathione -- one of the most potent detoxifiers for the liver. Bone broth and collagen powder are also excellent for this purpose.

Without sufficient amino acids, your liver can't complete phase 2 detoxification (the phase that actually excretes toxins), potentially making you more toxic. To avoid that pitfall, choose organic, pasture-raised, grass fed and finished meats, eggs from hens fed correctly, and wild-caught fish.

Keeping your liver clean and healthy is critical to a healthy life. Your liver has many functions: it is your body's main poison neutralizing organ; it balances hormones; boosts immunity; metabolizes fat; produces and stores your red blood cells.

You may notice that the shopping list from last week has no bread - not even gluten free, whole grain or sprouted breads; **no grains*** - not even oatmeal, quinoa or brown rice; and no dairy at all. Conventionally produced dairy has added hormones and antibiotics and will just add to the toxic load. Dairy is one of the most common allergens. Wheat has been eliminated because it is also one of the most common allergenic foods. Food intolerances cause a cascade of health issues, including leaky gut, immune reactions, and chronic inflammation, which affect metabolism. By removing the biggest culprits—including gluten (wheat), dairy, soy, corn, peanuts, and sweeteners—many clients lose up to seven pounds in the first seven days.

Even *healthy* **whole grains and starchy carbs*** have been eliminated during this two-week detox period to allow your body to cleanse as thoroughly as possible. Also, fruits are limited to two per day as they are typically high in fructose, a sugar that is metabolized in the liver. Once you detox, you will find your taste for healthy foods increases. Junk food, fast food and processed foods will begin to taste terrible. We are retraining your taste buds. In case you were wondering, taste buds' normal life cycle is anywhere from 10 days to two weeks! So committing to these two detox weeks will go a long way to making the whole process so much easier.

***Please note** – if you are a young woman of child bearing age, especially if your periods are erratic, I caution you not to go too low in carbs so as not to cause Hypothalamic Amenorrhea. It is important to get to a healthier weight, but not at the expense of your health and fertility. The other caution would be if you have adrenal fatigue. We would then adjust the plan for you when we coach. I have provided a link to an article by Dr. Lara Briden which will explain in detail about Hypothalamic Amenorrhea. She is a great resource if your periods are not regular.

Here's the basic plan, with details and explanations included, for these next two weeks (Don't worry—I'll also provide a streamlined version at the end of this chapter):

You will be eating:

- ✓ clean protein;
- ✓ non-starchy vegetables (unlimited);

✓ two fruit servings—*but no dairy or grains (even healthy whole grains, beans or starchy vegetables);*
✓ two tbsp. healthy fat

Eating your meals at regularly scheduled intervals (I call it eating structured, rhythmic meals) keeps your body working most efficiently and keeps you from getting so hungry you decide to ditch it all and eat whatever you can get your hands on! So, here's how the plan will look for the next two weeks:

Breakfast:

Upon rising, drink 16 oz. of pure water.

Measure out your salt allotment (1/4 tsp. for each 32 oz. of water consumed) and use it in your foods or put in your water during the day.

Here's where you can take your CLA if you choose to use it. Usually you take three 1,000 mg. soft gels daily, so you can take one before each meal or one before breakfast and two before dinner or all three before breakfast as I do, if you prefer.

Thirty minutes later have eight ounces of warm water into which you squeeze the juice of ½ of a lemon and, if you can tolerate it, a few sprinkles of cayenne pepper. This is a great liver cleanser and stimulates your bile production. Sip this.

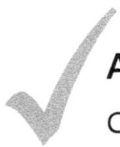

ANN'S PERSONAL TIP:

Cilantro is a very effective detoxifier and removes heavy metals from your body. When I periodically do a detox, I steep some cilantro with my morning tea for additional detoxification.

Breakfast options—alternate days or any combination you like, just eat your protein at each meal first:

Two or three eggs—scrambled, vegetable omelet*, over easy (in two teaspoons coconut or avocado oil-remember your allotment of fat for each day is two tablespoons);

use spices and herbs liberally and you can also have a cup of whatever tea you like sweetened with stevia or Lakanto, which are natural sweeteners that have no calories; or

A whey protein smoothie. If you prefer to use pea, hemp, collagen, cranberry or rice protein powders, that's fine as well. You can put one serving of fruit in the smoothie (six strawberries, eight cherries, 1/3 cup of frozen chopped mango or blueberries, one medium banana, ½ an avocado).

Some additional add-ins that bump up nutrition are: fresh or thawed frozen, organic spinach I've squeezed dry (spinach increases protein synthesis), some sprouts, broccoli, and even fresh flat leaf parsley or cilantro if I have it in the house. If you have a heavy duty blender, you can add a stalk of celery and a handful of any organic greens (kale, chard, arugula, Romaine) you like. Those all bump up the nutritional value and especially with the berries, you barely know they are there.

Ground flax, hemp or chia seeds, as well as sunflower and pumpkin seeds, are also a good addition and increase healthy fat and fiber content.

You can also add a scoop of a good green food to your smoothie, which will increase the protein and give you chlorophyll, which is a great detoxifier on its own. Instead of using water or coconut or almond milk for my smoothies, I use cooled herbal or green tea.

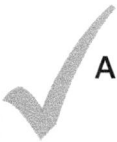

ANN'S PERSONAL TIP:

I call it an "omelet," but mine is more like a frittata – I soften the chopped veggies in my coconut or avocado oil and then add in the eggs that have been beaten, and once it is fairly set, I pop it under the broiler to finish cooking the top. You can also add a bit of real cheese on top if you like **after** the detox weeks and you have no problem with dairy.

If you have no health issues that would prevent you from using raw eggs, I sometimes blend 16 ounces of low sodium V-8 juice, one tablespoon of Brewer's yeast, one scoop collagen powder, one tablespoon Super Greens powder, two raw Omega-3 or pastured eggs, and one to two teaspoons ground black pepper until frothy for a quick, low calorie, alkalizing, high protein breakfast alternative. Studies show the black pepper stunts fat cell development and growth.

If you choose to take the digestive enzyme and probiotic—take them with the first few bites of whichever meals you use them with. If you only take them with one meal, I suggest it be dinner.

Water: When you figure out how many ounces of water you should be drinking daily, be sure to have 16 ounces before each meal (research has shown that drinking 16 ounces of water all at once, 15-30 minutes before a meal, increases metabolism by 30%) and throughout the day with your fiber and other supplements.

For example—let's say you weigh 180 pounds. You should shoot for at least 90 ounces of water daily. That's a little more than five 16 ounce servings - one before each meal and two more throughout the day. I also recommend ¼ teaspoon of natural, unprocessed salt for every 32 ounces of water you drink. So in this example, that would be ¾ teaspoon of salt. Try not to drink *while* you eat as it dilutes digestive enzymes.

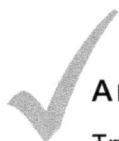

ANN'S PERSONAL TIP: ─────────────────────────

Try drinking eight ounces of hot water after your meals. It is believed to emulsify fat and help with digestion. You can steep a piece of fresh ginger in your cup and that will also help with digestion. My brother adds a few drops of liquid cayenne to his – the spice will help boost metabolism!

As I will explain below, I find it is better to limit your eating to just your meals. However, many people are used to eating more frequently throughout the day and find it easier to include snacks. So if that describes you, you can have a mid-morning snack here (list of options at the end).

Lunch:

Have 16 ounces of water and your CLA, if you use it, 30 minutes before lunch.

If you are using the fiber supplement with lunch, take it at least 30 minutes after your CLA with eight ounces of water at least 10 minutes before eating.

This is why I like to take my CLA first thing in the morning and my fiber before dinner. Then the fiber will not absorb the CLA, rendering both useless.

Aim for four ounces of a clean protein source from the list (if you are a man or a very physically active person, you can increase the protein to six ounces) and a salad or cooked vegetables.

Some lunch meal examples are:

A chicken burger (no bun) either sitting on a grilled Portobello or topped with sautéed baby bella mushrooms, steamed broccoli or zoodles with garlic and olive oil or organic tomato sauce; a salmon burger topped with roasted organic grape tomatoes and black olives; a roasted chicken thigh or breast on a big, green salad dressed with raw, organic apple cider vinegar and extra virgin olive or hemp oil.

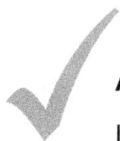

✓ ANN'S PERSONAL TIP: ————————————————

I boil, strain and puree a cup or two of lentils at a time and then portion the puree into ice cube trays and freeze. Then I pop them into a freezer bag and have individual portions that defrost quickly any time I decide to make burgers (or meatloaf or meatballs). Use these only after the detox weeks, of course. An added benefit is that some studies are showing lentils can help reduce dangerously high blood pressure levels!

https://www.express.co.uk/life-style/health/451062/Lentils-are-key-to-beating-high-blood-pressure

I do suggest you have at least one raw salad daily*, whether at lunch or dinner. Apple cider vinegar and flax seed, avocado, chia, hemp or extra virgin olive oil and whatever seasoning you like make a great dressing. I like the Bragg's Nutritional Yeast Seasoning and Organic Sea Kelp Delight Seasoning on my salads. Remember, limit the oil to two tablespoons a day for now; you can use one on your salad and one to cook your eggs and veggies. Don't stress if you use a little more healthy fat as long as you are avoiding the grains and starchy carbs for now.

*Have raw salad or just raw vegetables like red pepper strips, cucumbers, celery, Jerusalem artichoke or whatever you like ANYTIME. However, having the raw salad or even a combination that includes cooked and raw vegetables with dinner will help boost your fat burning and cleansing. The raw vegetables are loaded with enzymes that help you digest them and boost metabolism. But if you prefer to have them with lunch—go for it—just be sure to include them.

You can have a mid-afternoon snack between lunch and dinner *or* save it for an after-dinner snack as long as you don't eat after 7:00 pm, *if you find you need to snack.*

Dinner options:

Have 16 ounces of water and your last CLA 30 minutes before the dinner meal unless you took all three before breakfast.

Wait at least 30 minutes before you have your fiber supplement with at least eight ounces of water and wait 10 minutes before eating. You can take the fiber before any meal, but I find it most effective before the biggest meal of the day, which is usually dinner.

*When using a fiber supplement like Glucomannan, wait at least 30 minutes before taking any of your other supplements, especially any oil based supplements like CLA, vitamins D or E or fish oil, as the fiber will absorb them. It is best to take it separately from other supplements.

Dinners, especially for these next two weeks, will pretty much be the same as lunches. Play with the proteins and flavors and make your vegetable side dishes different so you don't get bored. If you have a big raw salad for lunch, you can have some cooked vegetables with dinner.

Snacks:

One of our goals in this plan is to switch over from being a sugar burner to becoming a fat burner. One effective strategy is to stop snacking between meals because every time you eat, you spike your insulin levels, which prevents fat burning and encourages fat storage. *Eating between meals creates insulin resistance, so I strongly suggest cutting out snacks and just eating properly structured meals.*

While some snacks are certainly healthy, and I will provide a list below, we often find ourselves mindlessly reaching for whatever's at hand, whether we are truly hungry or not.

The trick to eliminating the snacking habit is by adding, not subtracting, food from your diet. The absolute best way to quit mindlessly snacking is to stack your diet with protein, especially in the early hours. So a protein rich breakfast, as the plan provides, is a huge key. Protein increases satiety, which pacifies ghrelin, your body's primary hunger hormone. When you feel satiated, you won't want to reach for those snacks, making the habit much easier to break.

By including clean protein, healthy fat and fiber at each meal you will naturally be curbing hunger. However, some people find it difficult to go without a small snack and just do better having a mid-morning and either mid-afternoon or after dinner snack. As long as it is small and from the list below *and* you don't eat after 7 pm, you can do so.

- ✓ Be sure you are drinking your entire water allotment throughout the day; herbal teas are allowed at any time so if you are really hungry, a cup of tea and even bone broth may be just enough.
- ✓ You can have a piece or serving of fruit if you didn't use it in a smoothie (eight cherries, six-strawberries, one apple, pear, peach, nectarine or orange, ½ grapefruit, two plums or Clementines, 1/3- 1/2 cup of berries like blueberries, raspberries or fresh grapes; ½ cup of natural, unsweetened, organic applesauce.)
- ✓ Raw vegetables are a great choice between meals and they're unlimited! They add no calories and lots of fiber, vitamins and minerals.
- ✓ A hard-boiled egg, if you didn't have your eggs for breakfast – or even if you did. They make a great high protein, low fat snack.
- ✓ 10 almonds, walnuts, pecans or ½ cup of pistachios.
- ✓ 10 olives.
- ✓ You can combine your nuts with a piece of your fruit for the day or a piece of fruit with an ounce of a real, high quality cheese, if you eat dairy, *after the detox weeks*.
- ✓ A cup of broth or vegetable soup - you certainly can make it from scratch or buy a high quality, low sodium brand like Pacific Foods, Imagine Foods or Kitchen Basics that does not have any MSG - just be sure it is clear and not a cream soup. An excellent choice is bone broth. It is extremely healing to the digestive system, joints and skin, and the collagen helps with weight loss.

- ✓ One bottle of Beyond Organic Suero Viv (fermented whey beverage) or Kombucha.
- ✓ Frozen grapes - one cup.

This is our basic meal plan for the first two detox weeks. Once you complete those first two weeks, we will add in other foods gradually and carefully.

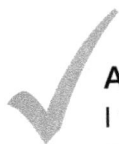

Ann's Personal Tip —————————————————————

I find it easiest to cook all my lunches on the weekend and have them ready to go. I also prefer to have the same thing each day. It's sort of "automating" the meals. It takes the guess-work out of the process and research seems to indicate it increases your chances of losing weight.

*Be sure to weigh yourself once each week and keep track of your meals, snacks, water intake and how you feel in your food log DAILY.

**You can go to the next chapter or go to Section Three and begin Spirit and Soul Detox or you can wait to do that when you are ready. Whatever works best for you is fine.

PROTEIN

Four ounces of high quality, organic (grass fed/finished, pasture raised, wild caught) protein at each meal. Skinless free range poultry— chicken, turkey; wild caught fish— salmon, tuna, sardines, mackerel, herring, flounder, sole, cod; ground chicken, turkey, bison, lean grass-fed beef, veal or lamb; chicken sausage (Al Fresco and Aidells are two good brands); Natural Choice or Applegate Naturals cold cuts (no nitrates or nitrites) occasionally; Eggs—Omega-3 or cage free, organic, if possible; whey, hemp, collagen, pea or rice protein powder

WATER

One-half your body weight ounces of water daily and teaspoon natural, unprocessed salt for every ounces of water

HERBS & SPICES:

Liberally. Black pepper, cinnamon, ginger, garlic, cayenne pepper, fennel, dill, turmeric, coriander, cumin, sage, rosemary, chili powder

UNLIMITED NON-STARCHY VEGETABLES

Particularly leafy greens, sprouts, herbs and all other green vegetables. Fresh or frozen organic chopped spinach (this is a great, fast addition to omelets, smoothies and burgers); Romaine, red and green leaf and whatever lettuces you love; artichokes, parsley, cilantro, kale, tomato, broccoli, cabbage, cauliflower, cucumbers, Brussels sprouts, eggplant, bell peppers, Swiss chard, mushrooms, squash (zucchini, yellow summer), celery, sprouts (alfalfa, broccoli), arugula, radicchio, broccoli rabe, broccolini, collard greens, escarole, endive, onions, garlic, green beans, radishes, watercress, asparagus; low sodium V-8 Juice

TEAS

Green, black, white, yerba mate, hibiscus, matcha, oolong, Rooibos, Tulsi and herbal teas

RAW, ORGANIC APPLE CIDER VINEGAR OR BALSAMIC

FAT

Two or three tablespoons of healthy fat daily. Extra virgin olive oil, virgin coconut oil*, avocado, hemp, flax seed oil; MCT oil, pasture butter, organic ghee; olives, avocadoes; unsalted, organic, raw nuts and seeds like almonds, macadamias, walnuts, cashews, pine nuts, chestnuts, pistachios, and sesame/ chia/flax/hemp/ pumpkin/ sunflower seeds

FRUIT

Two servings of fresh or frozen organic fruits daily. Apples (especially Granny Smith), bananas, avocado, mangoes, oranges, pineapple, lemons, grapefruit, cherries, strawberries, blueberries, raspberries, blackberries, pears, peaches

NATURAL SWEETENERS

No Sugar. You may use stevia, Lakanto or erythritol for sweetening.

NO DAIRY,

grains, starchy carbs (potatoes, corn, beets, winter squashes, sweet potatoes), no beans, legumes or sugar

WEEKS THREE & FOUR (AND BEYOND)
NOURISH/FUEL YOUR BODY

Congratulations for completing the first two detox weeks. I realize they are a challenge for some people who are used to eating a lot of carbs or just whatever they feel like having whenever the urge strikes! Things get easier from this point on because we will be adding in healthy, complex carbs and making your meals even more interesting and satisfying. We will apply this key to spirit and soul as well in Section three—but let's begin with body—the basic food plan.

Did you know that eating cheeseburgers, fries and sugary snacks all the time makes people gain weight? I can almost hear your response: well, duh—that's pretty obvious! Those foods cause you to gain weight but not only for the reason you may think. Yes, they are high (empty) calorie foods, but research by Washington University found that eating a high (bad) fat, high sugar diet changes the balance of bacteria in your gut and basically "programs" people's digestive systems to make them fat!

Nearly 40% of adults and 19% of youth are obese, the highest rate the country has ever seen, according to research released by the National Center for Health Statistics. Our food choices and the habits we create are critical to our overall health. The responsibility for our health rests solely with each one of us.

The temple in the Old Testament had specific gates and 2 Chronicles 23:19 tells us doorkeepers were stationed at the gates so no one unclean could enter! Once you cleanse your temple, (which you've just done!) you do not want to allow anything impure to enter. In Numbers 5:1-3 Moses was to send anyone who was unclean in any way outside the camp and so must we guard our "gates" (our heart, eyes, ears, nose, skin, mouth) and be very mindful and careful about what we allow to enter our temples. They either provide true nourishment or they are "empty" calories.

The concept here is similar to programming your computer—garbage in/garbage out; we can say—life in/life out or death in/death out. We decide! Deuteronomy 30:19 tells us to choose life!

First, I'd like to lay out the four basics for structuring your meals (and explain why). Then, I'll give you specifics breaking it down meal by meal so you know exactly what to do.

Rule One is choose nutrient-dense, fresh, one-ingredient, whole foods in the form closest to how God created them. These are the high quality, properly grown/raised, whole, one-ingredient foods I talked about in weeks one and two.

We will be creating meals around the freshest, whole, nutrient-dense foods available. I understand that buying all organic may not fit your budget. That's ok. The way I approach it is this: it is all about the choices you make on a daily basis. Make the best choices you can. So, first, in case you aren't sure—"nutrient-dense" foods are those foods that have a high nutrient-to-calorie ratio—they are rich in nutrients and relatively low in calories. Here think clean protein, fresh (or frozen) fruits and vegetables, legumes and whole grains. The opposite are "empty-calorie" or "energy-dense" foods—they are low (or totally lacking) in nutrition and high in calories. Here think fast foods, packaged, processed foods—and honestly I use the word lightly—I don't really consider most of them to be "food" at all. Basically they fill your belly but starve you at the cellular level. Many overweight and obese people are actually malnourished, as shocking as that may seem.

Here's a perfect example: Let's compare three ounces of potato chips to a three ounce baked potato. The baked potato has 80 calories as well as vitamins C, B6, fiber and potassium, while the chips provide a whopping 450 calories, 62% of which comes from unhealthy trans-fat!

Rule Two is to combine and prepare your foods carefully.

We will be combining foods and meals in ways that increase their nutritional value even more. While raw food enthusiasts would have you eating every meal raw, I'm not asking you to do that—I don't think it's practical for most people. In fact, the healthy compounds in certain vegetables are made more available to your body when they are cooked. For example, cooking tomatoes and combining them with a small amount of healthy fat like extra virgin olive oil or avocado oil makes the carotenoids and other important nutrients they contain easier for your body to use. So, drizzle a touch of olive oil on your tomato sauce to get the most benefit!

Cooking your carrots whole and cutting them up after cooking preserves much more of the nutritional value they contain. If they are organic, don't even peel them as most of the nutrients live right under the skin. Just scrub them well and serve these with a healthy fat source as well.

Combine iron rich foods like spinach, beets, eggs, chicken, turkey and sardines with a vitamin C rich food like lemon or lime, red or green bell peppers or salsa.

I encourage you to eat a raw salad daily. However, what you put on that salad can exponentially increase the nutritional content. A source of healthy fat makes your salad even healthier. Top with a few avocado slices, olives, some nuts or seeds or make a simple oil and vinegar dressing using flax, extra virgin olive, hemp, pumpkin seed, walnut or macadamia nut oil and raw, organic apple cider vinegar. Stay within your fat allotment—but use that fat wisely to get the most bang for your nutritional buck! Avoid bottled salad dressings made with inflammatory Omega-6 vegetable oils.

Also be aware that certain cruciferous vegetables like cabbage, broccoli, cauliflower and Brussels sprouts contain "goitrogenic" compounds that when eaten raw can depress thyroid function in sensitive people. If you have an underactive thyroid, simply cook those vegetables. If you have an overactive thyroid, eating those vegetables raw may help balance your thyroid.

Make it your new habit to use spices and herbs liberally in all your meals. Research is proving daily how effective they are in preventing and fighting disease and improving your overall health. A half teaspoon of cinnamon daily can lower cholesterol and blood sugar levels. It's so easy to do— sprinkle some in your protein smoothie or on your oatmeal (yes, we will be adding oatmeal!) or put some in your coffee or tea. Spice up your eggs with black pepper, turmeric and paprika, chipotle seasoning or dill and fennel. Turmeric is being studied for its inflammation fighting properties. Get creative and your meals will not only be more delicious, you will be healthier. These spices, as well as black and cayenne pepper, cloves, cardamom, cumin, turmeric, cinnamon, ginger and mustard are also helpful in weight loss. They boost metabolism, fight inflammation, stabilize blood sugar and increase the nutritional value of foods they are used in.

Regardless of your cooking method, cook your food at lower temperatures. Cooking at very high temperatures (grilling, broiling) not only destroys vital nutrients, it also produces advanced glycation end products (AGES). That acronym says it all because these substances cause inflammation and aging, and inflammation has been shown to cause weight gain! If you are roasting or baking your food, simply extend the cooking time and lower the temperature.

Be careful what type of fats you use. You'll notice this plan is not a "fat free" plan because fats are a vital macronutrient your body needs—however, it needs the right type of fats. For cooking, you should *never* use polyunsaturated vegetable oils like canola, corn, safflower, sunflower and soybean oil. They easily combine with oxygen and become rancid. Because of this tendency, they degrade very easily.

The best, most stable fats for cooking are virgin coconut oil, organic pasture butter, ghee, avocado and macadamia nut oil because they withstand higher temperatures without damage to their chemical structures since they have high smoke points. Regular olive oil is also suitable for light sautéing or stir frying at moderate temperatures not above 400 degrees. Oils like extra virgin olive oil, flax oil, hemp seed oil, pumpkin seed oil and walnut oil should not be heated but used as condiments, in salad dressings or in smoothies. They are very healthy oils.

Properly prepare your grains by soaking them in pure water with a tablespoon of either plain yogurt, kefir, Amasai or apple cider vinegar in a covered container overnight on the counter. Simply drain and cook in fresh water as usual the next day. The nutrients will be more available to your body because you deactivate the phytates they contain. If you neglect this, the phytates will block you from absorbing minerals those grains contain.

Rule Three is to eat in a way that keeps your pH balanced and alkaline.

We will structure meals in a way that helps you maintain a healthy acid/alkaline (pH) balance. This is very important as excess acidity in the body:

- ✓ Puts a lot of stress on the regulatory systems to balance these pH levels;
- ✓ Prevents effective absorption of vitamins and minerals;
- ✓ Pulls vital minerals from bones and teeth to buffer excess acidity;
- ✓ Prevents your body from repairing damaged cells;
- ✓ Makes you more susceptible to illness and fatigue and makes it much more difficult to lose weight!
- ✓ When your system is constantly acidic, your body shuttles the excess acid into fat stores. Then your body doesn't easily release that fat since it is protecting you!
- ✓ Acid-alkaline balance is not as easy to understand as once thought. Foods that may make one person acidic may not necessarily have the same effect on another person since we're all biochemically

unique. However, you can help keep your pH balanced simply by adjusting your diet to include more vegetables, fruits and green foods; avoiding sugary, processed junk foods, soft drinks, artificial sweeteners and grain products; drinking adequate water and managing stress. The unprocessed salt contains minerals that will also alkalize your system.

Rule Four is to choose quality nutritional supplements.

Last, besides structuring your diet around clean, whole foods—in the form closest to how God created them—clean, lean protein, whole grains in moderation, (organic wherever possible) fruits, vegetables, nuts, seeds, healthy fat and clean water, I want to mention the importance of using quality nutritional supplements. Unfortunately our soils are so depleted that even organic produce is not what it used to be, so we must supplement wisely.

Basic, foundational supplements are vitamin/mineral (and/or green food); vitamin D; probiotics, digestive enzymes, fiber, and omega-3s. Recent research is showing that most of us are seriously deficient in Vitamin D and this vitamin (which is really a hormone) improves insulin sensitivity, is cancer protective and important for a healthy cardiovascular system.

Probiotics and digestive enzymes help your digestive system to function at peak performance. You digest your food efficiently getting all the nutritional value and keeping the good bacteria replenished protects your immune system as well.

Fiber sweeps toxins and fat from your body, keeps you regular, makes your body work harder to digest meals (using more calories) and lowers the glycemic index of those meals.

Omega-3 fats stabilize moods, reduce inflammation, keep your heart healthy, are critical to brain health and possess myriad other benefits. Most people get too many Omega-6 fats, and it is very important to improve the ratio of Omega-3 to Omega-6 fats to ensure health. Research confirms they help with weight loss, too.

Ok, those are the "basics;" here are the specifics for the remaining four weeks.

You will continue eating the same basic meals, *except* you can now *gradually and in moderation*, begin to add specific, complex carbohydrates as well as beans and legumes. Remember to eat your protein first at each meal. Here is a list of the *"friendly carbs"* you can now include:

- ✓ whole grain, sprouted whole grain or gluten free bread (one slice);
- ✓ one whole grain or gluten free tortilla;
- ✓ one sweet potato, baked russet potato or one cup roasted red or purple potato;
- ✓ ½ cup of beans or legumes (kidney, black, Adzuki, chick peas, pinto, lentils, peas);
- ✓ ½ cup of brown, black, green, red, Jasmine, Basmati or whole grain rice, whole grain pasta* or barley; ½ cup squash (acorn, butternut, Delicata, spaghetti);
- ✓ ½ cup old fashioned or steel cut oats (not instant oats), buckwheat, millet or quinoa.
- ✓ *Very occasionally I use whole wheat pastas as well as gluten-free (Banza Chick Pea Pasta) and multi-grain pastas (Barilla Plus), which are a source of protein and ALA Omega-3s - there are so many available now you should have no problem finding them. While they are allowed in the plan now, I would still make them an occasional treat.
- ✓ Also try making your rice, pasta, potatoes and any grains ahead, cooling overnight and reheating before eating – it increases the resistant starch, which lowers their glycemic index among other benefits (see the chapter on resistant starch in Section One).
- ✓ Well balanced meals that contain protein, non-starchy carbs, a whole grain or starchy carb and healthy fat are what we are shooting for. When you combine a carb—even a healthy, whole grain one—with protein and fat, it automatically lowers the glycemic load and your body doesn't convert it to sugar as quickly. This is what we want.

You can add one carb to either breakfast or lunch each day beginning this week. It will look something like this:

Breakfast

Upon rising, drink 16 ounces of pure water; measure out your salt allotment. If you don't like the taste of it in your water, include it in your meals throughout the day.

You can take your CLA now if you choose to use it. Usually you take three 1,000 mg. soft gels daily, so you can take one before each meal or one before breakfast and two before dinner if you prefer, or all three before breakfast, which is what I do.

A few minutes later you can have eight ounces of warm water into which you squeeze the juice of ½ lemon and, if you can tolerate it, a few sprinkles of cayenne pepper. This is a great liver cleanser and stimulates your bile production. Sip this.

Before your actual breakfast, have whichever fiber supplement you prefer unless you choose to have your fiber before dinner only, which is fine. You must usually take fiber with at least eight ounces of water so just give yourself 10 minutes or so before you eat. (*Wait at least 30 minutes before taking any of your other supplements—especially oil based supplements like CLA fish oil—as the fiber will absorb them.)

Breakfast options—alternate days or any combination you like:

- ✓ two or three eggs—scrambled, vegetable omelet, sunny side up or over easy (in coconut or avocado oil or butter), soft or hard-boiled; or
- ✓ one or two chicken sausages;
- ✓ use spices and herbs liberally and you can also have a cup of whatever tea you like sweetened with stevia or Lakanto, which are natural sweeteners that have no calories; or
- ✓ a whey protein smoothie.

Here's the change: You can also have ½ cup of quinoa, millet, barley, buckwheat or oatmeal or one slice of bread; or one tortilla with the egg breakfast or the smoothie.

If you choose to take the digestive enzyme and probiotic—take them just before the first few bites of whichever meals you use them with. If you only take them with one meal, I suggest it be dinner.

Water: When you figure out how many ounces of water you should be drinking daily, be sure to have 16 ounces before each meal (remember drinking 16 ounces of water all at once before a meal increases metabolism by 30%) and throughout the day with your fiber and other supplements. Continue adding the appropriate amount of natural unprocessed salt—¼ teaspoon for every 32 ounces of water.

You can have a mid-morning snack here (list of options at the end) *if you choose to.*

Lunch options:

Have 16 ounces of water and your CLA, if you use it, 30 minutes before lunch.

At least 30 minutes after the CLA you can have the fiber supplement you've chosen (if using) with eight ounces of water and wait at least 10 minutes before eating.

Aim for four ounces of a clean protein source (if you are a man or a very active person, you can increase the protein to (six ounces) and a salad or cooked vegetables. (Refer back to the lunch options from the detox weeks with the following possible addition).

If you did NOT have one of the friendly carbs for breakfast today, choose one of these with your lunch:

- ✓ one slice of whole grain, gluten free or sprouted bread; or
- ✓ one whole grain or gluten free tortilla; or
- ✓ ¼-½ cup peas, beans, brown or whole grain rice, whole grain pasta, barley, millet, buckwheat, winter squash or quinoa; or
- ✓ one sweet or russet potato baked, or one cup roasted or boiled red or purple potatoes.

It may seem strange to eat your burger without a bun—but you could grill a Portobello mushroom and put your burger on it. Or, if you choose to have your carb for lunch, you can put your burger on a slice of whole grain bread and eat it open-face style.

Continue to have at least one raw salad daily, whether at lunch or dinner. Apple cider vinegar and flax seed, hemp seed, avocado or extra virgin olive oil and whatever seasoning you like make a great dressing. Continue to keep the oil to two or three tablespoons a day—you can split them between your salad and cooking your eggs or veggies.

You can have a mid-afternoon snack between lunch and dinner or save it for an after dinner snack, *if you still choose to,* as long as you don't eat after 7:00 pm.

Dinner options:

Have 16 ounces of water and your last CLA 30 minutes before the dinner meal unless you took all three before breakfast. Then have your fiber supplement with 16 ounces of water and wait 20-30 minutes before eating.

Dinners will remain the same as the detox weeks. Play with the proteins and flavors and make your vegetable side dishes different so you don't get bored. If you have a big raw salad for lunch, have some cooked veggies with dinner.

Snack options:

Be sure you are drinking your entire water allotment throughout the day; herbal teas are allowed at any time so if you are really hungry, a cup of tea or bone broth may be just enough.

The snacks are the same as the first two weeks. You may also choose to include an ounce of a high quality, raw cheese if you include dairy.

Pay attention to your body:

As you add in the friendly carbs this week, very gradually and moderately—pay attention to how they make you feel—note it in your journal. Do any upset your stomach? Make you gassy? Feel fatigued after you eat them? Take note and substitute a different one next time and see if the result is different.

I also encourage you to sit down and eat your meals peacefully and mindfully, savoring each bite. Enjoy the textures and flavors. Eat slowly and chew your food thoroughly—digestion begins in your mouth! Begin your meals with a prayer of thanks to God.

Also, after this week note whether you still lost weight. I suggest only adding in the carbs early in the day at this stage to allow your body to adjust. You are much more likely to be active enough to burn them off if you have them earlier in the day.

*Be sure to weigh yourself once each week and keep track of your meals, snacks, water intake and how you feel in your food log DAILY.

**You can go directly to the next chapter or skip over to Section Three and begin spirit and soul nourish and fuel. You can follow along doing the weeks that pertain to the body and the spirit and soul at the same time or focus just on the body first. You can wait and do the spirit and soul weeks after you finish the part of the plan that addresses the body or incorporate it as you go along. Whatever works best for you is fine.

PROTEIN

Four ounces of high quality, organic (grass fed/finished, pasture raised, wild caught) protein at each meal. Skinless free range poultry—chicken, turkey; wild caught fish—salmon, tuna, sardines, mackerel, herring, flounder, sole, cod; ground chicken, turkey, bison, lean grass-fed beef, veal or lamb; chicken sausage (Al Fresco and Aidells are two good brands); Natural Choice or Applegate Naturals cold cuts (no nitrates or nitrites) occasionally; Eggs—Omega-3 or cage free, organic, if possible; whey, hemp, collagen, pea or rice protein powder

WATER

One-half your body weight in ounces of water daily and ¼ teaspoon natural, unprocessed salt for every 32 ounces of water

TEAS

Green, black, white, yerba mate, hibiscus, matcha, oolong, Rooibos, Tulsi and herbal teas

HERBS & SPICES:

Use liberally. Black pepper, cinnamon, ginger, garlic, cayenne pepper, fennel, dill, turmeric, coriander, cumin, sage, rosemary, curry, chili powder

UNLIMITED NON-STARCHY VEGETABLES

Particularly leafy greens, sprouts, herbs and all other green vegetables. Fresh or frozen organic chopped spinach (this is a great, fast addition to omelets, smoothies and burgers); Romaine, red and green leaf and whatever lettuces you love; artichokes, parsley, cilantro, kale, tomato, broccoli, cabbage, cauliflower, cucumbers, Brussels sprouts, eggplant, bell peppers, Swiss chard, mushrooms, squash (zucchini, yellow summer), celery, sprouts (alfalfa, broccoli), arugula, radicchio, broccoli rabe, broccolini, collard greens, escarole, endive, onions, garlic, green beans, radishes, watercress, asparagus; low sodium V-8 Juice

BEANS/LEGUMES

1/4-1/2 cup beans or legumes
Lentils, peas, black/red kidney/pink/ garbanzo/cannellini, Adzuki beans

FRIENDLY COMPLEX CARBS

Whole grain, sprouted whole grain or gluten free bread (one slice); one whole grain or gluten free tortilla; one sweet potato, baked russet potato or one cup roasted red or purple potato; ½ cup of brown, black, green, red, Jasmine, Basmati or whole grain rice, whole grain pasta or barley; ½ cup squash (acorn, butternut, Delicata, spaghetti); ½ cup old fashioned or steel cut oats, buckwheat, millet or quinoa

FAT

Two or three tablespoons of healthy fat daily. Extra virgin olive oil, virgin coconut oil*, avocado, hemp, flax seed oil; MCT oil, pasture butter, organic ghee; olives, avocadoes; unsalted, organic, raw nuts and seeds like almonds, macadamias, walnuts, cashews, pine nuts, chestnuts, pistachios, and sesame/ chia/flax/hemp, pumpkin

FRUIT

Two servings of fresh or frozen organic fruits daily. Apples (especially Granny Smith), bananas, avocado, mangoes, oranges, pineapple, lemons, grapefruit, cherries, strawberries, blueberries, raspberries, blackberries, pears, peaches

Natural Sweeteners

No Sugar. May use Stevia, Lakanto, or Erythritol for sweetening tea

RAW, ORGANIC APPLE CIDER VINEGAR OR BALSAMIC

WEEK FIVE:
INTENTIONAL EXERTION - EXERCISE

You knew we would get to this eventually—you cannot be truly healthy unless you are active and exercise is essential for releasing fat and getting a fit, strong body. We've all heard the phrase "use it or lose it" and it is true. Muscle that is not used atrophies and shrinks. If you've ever seen someone who's broken a bone—leg or arm—when the cast finally came off, not only was the skin pale and pasty looking, but you could clearly see how much muscle was lost.

If you need to be convinced of the value of adding daily exercise, here are my top 10 reasons to exercise:

#1: Exercise burns calories

You need to burn more calories than you consume in order to lose weight. Regular exercise uses up those excess calories and sugar that would otherwise be stored as fat.

#2 Exercise increases energy

Regular physical activity increases your stamina by boosting the body's production of energy-promoting neurotransmitters. It also provides oxygen to your cells which is necessary in energy production.

#3 Exercise helps boost your mood

Working out has been proven to help regulate mood; it is an excellent way to manage stress and reduce anxiety by releasing feel-good brain chemicals called endorphins.

#4 Exercise boosts metabolism

When you diet alone, you lose "weight" and the scale will move. However, you lose water and muscle that way, not fat. The more muscle you have the higher your metabolism and the more calories you burn—all the time. Exercise builds and preserves muscle and helps you burn fat, which is what your goal should be.

#5 Exercise improves your body composition

When you gain muscle and lose fat you might not see a huge drop on the scale, but your clothes will begin to fit better. You might release three pounds of fat and gain two pounds of lean muscle and the scale may only show a one pound "weight loss." In reality, you made a five pound improvement in your body's composition.

#6 Exercise creates momentum

One healthy habit naturally leads to another. When you make a positive change, such as exercising regularly, you tend to naturally work on other health improvements as well, such as improving your diet, managing stress and getting adequate rest.

#7 Exercise lowers insulin levels

Elevated insulin levels are not only the main cause of diabetes (which has reached epidemic proportions in our country), but also of high cholesterol, triglycerides and blood pressure! You can not only control the symptoms associated with these conditions, but in many cases actually reverse them totally. The only side-effects are energy and improved overall fitness and health, unlike the drugs that might be prescribed.

#8 Exercise improves your brain

Studies have found that regular exercise can reduce your risk of Alzheimer's and even boost your brainpower. Increasing oxygen and blood flow nourishes the brain, and exercise is the best way to do that. Good physical health is important for good brain function.

#9 Exercise helps improve your sleep

If you are struggling with insomnia or other sleep problems, regular exercise can help you enjoy a much better night's sleep. Just don't exercise too close to bedtime.

#10 Exercise boosts your immune system

Moderate exercise has been linked to a positive immune system response and a temporary boost in the production of the cells that attack bacteria. During moderate exercise, immune cells circulate through the body more quickly and are better able to kill bacteria and viruses. Regular, consistent exercise can lead to substantial, cumulative benefits in immune system health over the long-term.

Exercising at moderate intensity for 450 minutes per week (just over an hour a day) lowered the risk of premature death by 39%, compared to non-exercisers.

I hope you are convinced! However, if you haven't exercised in years, you must check with your healthcare practitioner to be sure you are able to begin an exercise program safely. The easiest way to get exercise and a way almost everyone can do is to begin walking. You can walk in your home, on a treadmill, around the block or on a trail.

We can all agree too much stress is bad for your health. But did you know it can even affect your waistline and fitness performance? In a Yale study, scientists found stress was associated with poor muscle recovery after a workout, even when correcting for fitness level and training experience.

https://www.ncbi.nlm.nih.gov/pubmed/22688829

Something as simple as taking 10 minutes each day to relax and unwind can make all the difference. For example, take a break in the middle of the day for a quiet walk outside with no phone; meditate at home after work or listen to relaxing music during your coffee break or drive home. Just taking a few minutes per day will boost your mood and improve your mental and physical health in addition to making your exercise efforts more effective.

There is a fine line here. You need rest and you need activity. Sitting for long periods of time – even if you regularly exercise – is as dangerous to your health as smoking! You don't want to be "actively sedentary," which scientist Katy Bowman describes as:

"Actively sedentary is a new category of people who are fit for one hour but sitting around the rest of the day... You can't offset 10 hours of stillness with one hour of exercise."

I suggest setting a timer on your phone or FitBit so you can remember to get up every 30-40 minutes and move! Being sedentary has also been shown to increase anxiety and high mortality rates.

The cure isn't just exercising more—*it is sitting less.* For every 30 minutes of sitting, it is recommended you move for a minimum of 1 minute and 45 seconds. Stretch, walk around, do a few squats, wall pushups, high knees, march in place, lunges or a 60 second wall sit! It gets blood circulating. Make every bathroom break a movement break as well! God designed our bodies to be active.

Standing desks are popular today, but if you can't invest in something like that right now, besides these activity breaks, consider sitting on an exercise ball or a balance disc for a few hours a day! You will be engaging core muscles while you sit.

Your goal is to work up to an additional 10,000 steps day (which is equivalent to 5 miles). Walking 10,000 additional steps most days of the week will boost your weight loss and fitness efforts greatly. At a minimum, while trying to release weight you should shoot for at least three days a week to begin with, preferably working up to five.

Here's an easy way to work up to the 10,000 steps: Begin by walking 1,000 extra steps. Increase that each day or every other day by 500 or 1,000 steps until you reach the goal of 10,000 steps at least three days a week and preferably five or six days a week.

Once you are comfortable with five miles most days a week, it is good to vary the routine so your body doesn't get so used to it. Your body is very intelligent (remember Who created it!). When you do the same workout routine, in exactly the same way, your body gets used to it—it adapts. When that happens, it becomes so efficient at doing that routine that you burn fewer calories. You want to vary your routine—the number of repetitions, speed, intensity and specific exercises every few weeks to keep your body surprised, and you will continue burning the maximum number of calories.

Dr. Timothy Miller, sports medicine specialist, advises: *"Don't do the same workout every day. Add something that makes your body work differently."*

Timing Is Everything

My suggestion is that you schedule your exercise sessions in the morning if at all possible. If you find it easier or more convenient to exercise in the afternoon or evening, by all means do so. Obviously the point is to just be sure to get up and do it every day.

The biggest advantage to scheduling exercise first thing in the morning is that you get it done before other things intrude and possibly cause you to put it off altogether. Consistency and compliance are keys. The more consistently you follow through and exercise, the more successful your efforts will be.

Exercising first thing in the morning, before breakfast, also allows you to tap into stored energy (fat!) and burn that as fuel rather than simply the meal you just ate. So that is another advantage to getting up a little earlier and exercising before you begin your day.

You will find also that you have so much more energy for the rest of your day; it's a wonderful way to manage stress and release endorphins, those feel-good brain chemicals. What a terrific way to begin your day on a positive note! You might even consider doing 30 minutes first thing in the morning and 30 minutes on your lunch hour or before dinner. That would also be a great way to schedule it for maximum results.

However, if you find it easier to schedule exercise later in the day, by all means do so. Just be sure not to exercise too close to bed time as it may make it more difficult for you to unwind and get to sleep.

Here's a bonus: Walking is a "weight bearing" exercise and research shows doing weight bearing exercise helps preserve and build bone, which is critical in preventing osteoporosis. It's estimated that one in three women will develop osteoporosis at some point in their lifetime (compared to one in 50 men), and osteoporosis is believed to be the leading degenerative disease in the developed world.

Walking is considered to be "cardio" or aerobic exercise and also weight bearing since the definition of that term is "any activity that requires you to stand up and support yourself." Here are some other "weight bearing" exercises you may want to include in your routine:

- ✓ Jogging or walking/jogging intervals
- ✓ Running/sprinting intervals
- ✓ Weightlifting (including using exercise bands, kettle bells, dumbbells or medicine ball)
- ✓ Boxing or kickboxing
- ✓ Rebounding (no impact on joints)
- ✓ Jumping rope

Depending on your fitness level, I suggest you also include two to three sessions of weight training, as well as the walking each week, in order to preserve/build muscle. Muscle burns fat and is more metabolically active than other tissue. When you have more lean muscle, your basal metabolic rate (BMR) is higher. In other words, even when lying in bed, doing nothing, your body burns more calories. That alone is a great incentive for building muscle!

You can do a workout using hand weights, exercise bands or even a medicine ball or kettle bells. However, you can begin with no equipment other than your own body. You can do wall sits, lunges and squats to develop your leg muscles and wall pushups and chair dips to develop your upper body.

If you work, you can even get short bursts of these body-weight exercises in the rest room periodically during the work day. Not only will you build muscle, but moving in this way throughout the day is extremely healthy for you and you'll be more clear headed as you increase oxygen and blood flow to the brain! The key when doing weight training is to do it every other day or work different parts of the body if you do it on consecutive days. Always take a day of rest between sessions to allow your muscles to repair.

Two good tips to increase the effectiveness of your workout are: think about and focus mentally on the muscle(s) you are working. It actually maximizes the effect and increases the benefit you gain. Thinking is a powerful and underused tool! Also, to increase your motivation—use visualization. A great way is to have a picture—either of how you used to look and want to look again or a picture from a magazine of how you want to shape your body. Put it where you can look at it daily—and put a few of your health confessions with it to speak as you look at the picture. It may sound strange—but it is a powerful motivator and you'd be surprised at how much this increases your resolve!

One caution: exercise is addictive. If you haven't exercised in a while, you may find that hard to believe—but it is true. You release endorphins—feel-good chemicals—and who doesn't like to feel good? While it is one of the better things you can become "addicted" to, exercising too much (overtraining) is counterproductive. If you spend hours on the treadmill each day, you actually are creating inflammation in your body which breaks it down rather than building it up. So be moderate—balance is key in all we do.

Additional Resources

Once you begin your exercise routine, if you are ready to shake it up and vary your routine, here are some great resources to pump up your walk!

I want to say a little about high intensity interval training (HIIT) which happens to be my exercise method of choice. It is also called burst training. It is a training technique in which you give all-out, 100% effort through quick, intense bursts of exercise, followed by short, sometimes active, recovery periods. This type of training gets and keeps your heart rate up and causes increased fat burning in less time. There are many different approaches and plenty of DVDs that you can use and I have some links to a few of my favorites on the Resources page.

Research reveals that HIIT can even stop aging at the cellular level. According to the study, HIIT does this by increasing the capacity of mitochondria. In addition, it rejuvenates the cells' ribosomes, which produce protein building blocks.

HIIT isn't the only type of exercise that can reverse aging. Strength training can make weak muscles stronger, decrease arthritis pain, improve memory, and prevent bone loss and even reverse age-related bone loss in men.

Leslie Sansone has excellent walking DVDs you can simply pop into your DVD player and use in the privacy of your own home—rain or shine. There are one-, two-, three-, four-, and five-mile workouts, as well as those that incorporate interval training, alternating walking and jogging, Pilates, kickboxing and also stretch band and hand weight exercises also incorporate weight training. You can do them at your own pace and work up to the more challenging routines. I use these myself when I can't walk outside, and I highly recommend them. The DVDs are available from Walmart, Target and other stores as well as through her website.

If you enjoy walking outdoors or on a treadmill, find some uplifting and motivating music to keep you moving.

There are so many ways to vary your routine once you get the habit set and improve your fitness level:

walk, play a sport, play with your children or grandchildren, take a class, ride a bicycle, dance, skate, rebound, use kettle bells, Pilates, tai chi, Zumba, qi gong, interval training, HIIT, jumping rope, weight training, exercise ball/bands, DVDs/tapes; functional fitness; PraiseMoves, the Christian alternative to yoga.

And if you feel like you just don't have a 30-minute block to exercise, here's some very good news: recent research shows physical exercise does not need to be done in bouts lasting at least 10 minutes to lower your risk of death. Those who got at least 30 minutes of moderate-to-vigorous physical activity per day, regardless of how it was accumulated, had a mortality risk that was one-third lower than those who remained sedentary. So the take-away is – even if you do 5 or 10 minute bursts of activity throughout the day, you will reap positive health benefits!

So there really is NO EXCUSE—the bottom line is: GET MOVING!!

*Be sure to weigh yourself once each week and keep track of your meals, snacks, water intake and how you feel in your food log DAILY.

**Remember you can go directly to the chapter in Section Three that deals with spirit and soul exercise at this point or save it for the end.

WEEK SIX
REST AND REBOOT

Adequate sleep and rest is critical not only for overall health, to consolidate memories and learning and to allow your organs to replenish and rejuvenate themselves, but for weight loss and fitness as well. Doctors are now acknowledging the fact that sleep disruption seriously affects the physical body in many ways, including causing weight gain.

We may not all need exactly the same number of hours to function optimally, but according to the National Sleep Foundation, most adults need between six and nine hours.

Studies have demonstrated that almost one-third of U.S. adults get less than six hours of sleep each day, which is associated with low-grade, chronic inflammation and worsening insulin resistance, as well as increased risk for obesity, Type 2 diabetes, and cardiovascular disease. Complete proteins like grass-fed, pasture raised animal meats, eggs or a quality protein shake will increase chemicals in the brain that improve sleep as well as your mood. This is all due to the amino acid tryptophan, which is a precursor to serotonin. The feel-good hormone - serotonin makes us feel happy and motivated throughout the day. Serotonin then turns into melatonin, which helps us sleep at night! Without that complete protein at the start of the day, this conversion can't take place, leaving you tired and moody. One more reason I strongly recommend starting your day with a source of clean protein.

Many scientists and researchers are finding that sleep deprivation may lead to overeating and weight gain because it increases levels of the appetite stimulating hormone ghrelin and decreases levels of leptin, a hormone that makes you feel full and satisfied. Could this be the missing piece of the puzzle as to why so many Americans who are chronically sleep-deprived can't seem to maintain a healthy weight?

Perhaps you've heard it said that the hours you sleep before midnight are even more important for health than those after. Research, as well as Chinese medicine, reveals that sleep between the hours of 10:00 pm and 6:00 am are more restorative than from 3:00 am to 11:00 am. The different organ systems in your body are repaired and restored during those hours of sleep. For example, the adrenals are replenished between 11:00 pm and 1:00 am. If you don't get to sleep until 3:00 am, they do not have the chance to be replenished. Also, melatonin, the hormone that helps you sleep, peaks between midnight and 1:00 a.m.

Besides adding to stress, depression and irritability, poor sleep habits have been linked to diabetes, obesity, reduced growth hormone release, increased inflammatory activity, as well as other health conditions.

So the first order of business is to be sure you are getting adequate, restful, restorative sleep each night.

It's important to go to sleep early enough, *when you're tired*, otherwise your body releases the stress hormone cortisol to keep you awake, which not only causes a stress response but makes it more difficult to fall asleep. This becomes a vicious cycle of being sleep deprived, overtired and stressed. You end up tired but wired and unable to sleep.

If you experience problems falling asleep or staying asleep, there could be several causes. Let's begin with your sleep environment.

I don't know about you, but when I walk into a space that's cluttered and messy, it's extremely agitating to me. Actually, many people find it difficult to relax and fall asleep in a messy, cluttered room. So, if that is an issue, you may need to begin by cleaning, decluttering and organizing your bedroom.

Next, make sure your mattress, pillows, sheets, blankets, and comforters are comfortable for you. One person prefers a firmer mattress and someone else, a softer one. You are the best judge of that for yourself. The mattress industry used to tell you to replace your mattress every eight to ten years, and later changed that to every five to seven years. Carefully examine your mattress and if it sags or looks worn anywhere, if there are any coils or wires visible or if it makes creaking or squeaking noises when you move around— take those as indications that you should start shopping around for a new mattress.

It's best to keep the temperature in your bedroom slightly on the cooler side rather than toasty warm. In general, the optimal temperature for sleep is on the cool side, between 60 and 68 degrees. Temperatures too far above or below this can lead to restlessness. Temperatures in this range help core body temperature to decrease which in turn initiates sleepiness. A growing number of studies are finding that temperature regulation plays a role in many cases of chronic insomnia. For troubled sleepers, a cool room and a hot-water bottle at the feet rapidly dilates blood vessels and therefore actually helps lower core temperature, which can push the internal thermostat to a better setting.

There are two schools of thought about whether you should have a TV in the bedroom or not as light, and particularly blue light from the TV and other electronics, can hinder the production of melatonin, the hormone that helps you sleep. Some experts say never watch TV and others say it's ok. Again, that is a personal choice. If you find watching TV stimulates you and prevents you from falling asleep, then obviously, stop doing it! The more completely dark the room is, the deeper and healthier your quality of sleep will be, the reason being there will be no light to hinder melatonin production. So, blackout shades or even a sleep mask, if it doesn't bother you, may be helpful.

Also it is helpful to buy an inexpensive pair of blue light blocking glasses from Amazon and wear them the last few hours before bedtime while you are watching TV or if you are on your computer, phone or other electronics to keep the blue light from stimulating your brain and hindering your ability to fall asleep. I use these and find they have made a huge difference for me.

Some people find a white noise machine to be very helpful. There are several different ones on the market (my husband and daughter use one made by Homedics), which you can easily find at department or drug stores as well as Walmart or Target. They create the sounds of a spring rain, heartbeat, white static-like noise, ocean waves or a mountain stream—soothing, calming sounds that cancel out any distracting noises. Even just running a fan works. Having a pre-bed ritual is also helpful, such as a warm bath or shower, reading something calming, listening to soft music, praying or meditating. Whole Tones Lullabies is especially soothing and calming music to play softly.

Actually a warm bath with Epsom salts or Magnesium flakes is an extremely relaxing way to prepare for a good night's sleep. I find Epsom salts with lavender oil in my Walmart. That's a great sleep inducing combination.

We have to mention food and drink here as well. The obvious things to avoid close to bedtime are caffeine (chocolate, coffee, teas except herbal ones, soda, energy drinks) and sugary, empty-calorie foods. However, very cold foods may also make your body work harder to bring them up to your body temperature and digest them. A raw salad is a wonderful food choice—but not just before bed! Eating fatty, protein foods too close to bedtime can also keep you up. Protein is important for health and weight loss; however, sticking to clean protein and not eating past 6 or 7 pm will help here. Protein is a stimulating food—it turns up your metabolism, remember? Well, that's a good thing, just not right before bedtime.

Good, sleep-enhancing foods would include whole grains like brown rice and quinoa, which also contain tryptophan, an amino acid that increases levels of calming brain chemicals and melatonin. Oats are another great whole grain choice. (You can have a small serving later in the day once you have reached your goal or if you have adrenal fatigue.) Legumes like peas and lentils with your evening meal once you reach your goal are also great because they digest very slowly. If you have difficulty falling asleep or staying asleep, it could indicate adrenal fatigue. Increasing your intake of minerals with a mineral supplement or green drinks and leafy green vegetables will help bump up your mineral intake. (The sea salt provides minerals as well.)

Herbal teas are a wonderful choice to help you relax and unwind in the evening. Chamomile is a classic choice, but any caffeine-free, herbal tea you enjoy would be great such as peppermint, Tulsi Sweet Rose, Rooibos, ginger, lemon, valerian, blueberry, or even a blend specifically formulated to relax you, like Celestial Seasonings Sleepy Time, Organic India Tulsi Sleep or Bigelow Benefits Sleep.

You may find a scoop of collagen powder, which is tasteless, in your tea helps with sleep. You may also choose to use a calcium-magnesium drink which is calming and relaxing. I usually combine that with a scoop of collagen powder. You can find links to the ones I use on the Resource and Links page on my website.

You may find aromatherapy to be helpful. You can use various essential oils, a few drops either in a diffuser, in your bath or on your pulse points. Lavender, ylang ylang and chamomile are some that are used for relaxation. You might put a few drops of lavender oil, for example, into some magnesium oil and apply to the soles of your feet before bedtime. Both have very calming and relaxing properties.

Bach Flower Remedies are a great tool for relieving stress and emotional imbalances in a very natural way, promoting calm and relaxation. You may also need to address underlying conditions such as adrenal fatigue or thyroid problems and even balance hormone levels. All these things can be accomplished naturally.

Taking time out to rest is also extremely important. This is giving your body that chance to reboot. By "rest or rebooting," I simply mean disconnecting from stresses of life for a time—even just 15-20 minutes a day. Consider it a mini-vacation! Scripture tells us Jesus off went off by Himself (Matthew 14:13, 23 and many other scriptures) as well as calling the disciples to come away by themselves (Mark 6:31). Here are a few suggestions for rebooting:

Several times throughout the day, close your eyes for a few minutes and breathe deeply and slowly. You'd be surprised how calming and refreshing that is. Most people are very shallow breathers. Practice progressive relaxation exercises that have you tense and then relax your muscles. Massage is also a nice way to break away from the routine. Take a praise and worship break periodically! Even five minutes will do wonders.

Pamper yourself. Employ all your physical senses: take a warm bubble bath scented with essential oils; use Bach flower essences or diffuse essential oils to create a relaxing atmosphere; prepare a special (hopefully healthy) treat and enjoy it; sit in the warm sunlight and enjoy the sensation on your skin. We are children of the Most High and without being arrogant or prideful, we should treat ourselves with the same care and respect as we would any other child of God. I've heard this concept called self-compassion, but the Bible calls it the Royal Law in James 2:8 and Galatians 5:14.

One of the absolute best ways to reboot is to take a nature break. A brisk walk outside, especially in the middle of your day, will get you recharged and ready to focus. If you work in a city or someplace where you can't get in nature, studies show even just looking at pictures of nature will boost creativity and activate the areas of the brain associated with productivity!

When your timer rings to remind you to get up and move – get in the habit of taking five slow, deep breaths. That will oxygenate your brain, give you a burst of energy and relieve stress.

A great way to give yourself a break and relieve stress is to color. Yes, I mean use colored pencils or crayons like your five-year-old does! There are a huge number of wonderful adult coloring books to choose from. Researchers suggest they are an effective alternative to meditating and can reduce anxiety, create focus and bring about more mindfulness. There are some beautiful coloring books that have scripture verses – that combines two effective methods of rebooting!

Don't think it's a waste of time to just sit quietly and daydream now and then! Disconnecting from the routine of the day with no other agenda can really refresh your outlook and boost productivity.

*Be sure to weigh yourself once each week and keep track of your meals, snacks, water intake and how you feel in your food log DAILY.

**It's important to rest and reboot your spirit and soul and you can go to the chapter in Section Three that addresses this whenever you are ready. Just don't forget about it!

Week Seven
Putting It All Together - Body

You already have the basic principles in place and by now they have become just about second nature! Let's just quickly review the basics and add a few "bump ups":

Protein

Eat some form of clean protein at each meal. Protein has the greatest thermic effect—bumps your metabolism up more than other nutrients. Protein at breakfast is especially important as it interrupts production of cortisol and gets your metabolism going.

BUMP UP: By including beans and legumes in your meals and in your burgers and soups, you increase fiber and plant protein and if you also add in some spinach, it increases protein synthesis—you get more protein bang for your nutritional buck! Just be aware of possible damage from lectins, particularly from beans, which I explained in Weeks One and Two.

Beans are a low glycemic food that have more fiber than any other vegetable, providing 20% of your daily requirement in just one serving; they're believed to lower pancreatic, prostate and colon cancer risk; block absorption of cancer causing toxins, and protect DNA from free radical damage; eating beans or lentils twice a week lowers breast cancer risk; and as little as 1/3 cup of black beans a day (delicious on a salad!) cuts heart attack risk by 40%! So don't be afraid to include a small amount of beans and legumes.

Water

Continue to drink at least one half your body weight in ounces of water daily and use ¼ teaspoon natural, unprocessed salt for every 32 ounces of water you consume. As you release excess fat, you will be naturally reducing the amount you drink. Remember, you can simply measure out the salt and be sure to use it in your food—or just put ¼ teaspoon into a few glasses of your water, which is what I do. By the way, you can still include salt in your food even if you use your allotment in your water.

I also like to add ½ teaspoon of a structured water to one or two of my water servings as it is a catalyst that increases nutrient assimilation and aids in detoxification. It also increases the alkalinity of the water. I will give you links for two of the ones I use on the resources page.

If drinking a lot of plain water is starting to become difficult, you can infuse your water with different herbs, fruits and veggies. They sell infuser water bottles and pitchers that have a separate well where you put the foods you are using to add flavor, making it so easy. You can certainly just put the fruit, herbs and/or veggies directly in your water bottle or glass and let them infuse directly. You can use lemon or lime wedges, cucumber slices, mint, blueberries, strawberries, orange slices, basil, pineapple, watermelon, cantaloupe, grapefruit, apples, rosemary, parsley, cilantro, thyme, cinnamon sticks, fresh ginger, cloves, vanilla bean or any combo of those or whatever speaks to you!

BUMP UP: Vary the water temperature for different results:

Cold water increases your metabolism. Your body has to work in order to warm it enough for you to be able to absorb it. First thing in the morning have a glass of cold water to get your metabolism pumping.

During the day, but not at mealtimes, alternate drinking a glass of ice cold water and then a cup of hot water. You will encourage your body's elimination processes and bump up calorie burn as well.

Hot water detoxifies your body, helps emulsify fats and also stimulates peristalsis, which helps your body eliminate wastes. This is why I suggested starting your day with eight ounces of hot/warm (not boiling) water to which you add the juice of half a lemon and a teaspoon of the fresh lemon zest. It will clean you out, detox you and keep your bowels moving. If you're really courageous, you can even add a sprinkle of cayenne pepper to stimulate bile flow and help cleanse your liver.

Lukewarm or room temperature water is an appetite suppressant. Fifteen to 30 minutes before a meal, down 16 ounces of room temperature water to suppress your appetite and boost metabolism. If you choose to use CLA, this is the time to take it.

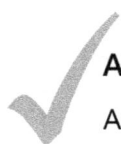

Ann's Personal Tip: —————————————————

Another way to use water is by ending your shower with 30 seconds of the coldest water you can stand hitting your neck and upper back. It will stimulate your brown fat which is active fat that keeps you lean. However, do not do this if you have any heart issues and definitely go from hot to warm to cool to cold gradually – never suddenly from hot to cold.

Fiber

Increase your fiber intake by increasing your intake of non-starchy vegetables—both cooked and raw—and you can also continue taking a fiber supplement before a meal. Fiber will help you stay regular, lower the glycemic index of the meal, make your body work harder to digest it, help you feel fuller; it will also reduce C-Reactive Protein, an inflammation marker, by 63%; and trap and sweep fat and toxins from your body.

Bump up: Try using Miracle Noodles which are made from Konjac root fiber. They are calorie free and pure fiber! They do not taste like regular pasta, but if you need something on one of those "hungry days" and don't want to ruin your efforts—add a package of Miracle Noodles into some bone broth or a non-cream based vegetable or bean soup. It's filling, satisfying and a truly free food! Also add ground flax, hemp or chia seeds to your smoothies to boost fiber and healthy fat.

Meal Composition

The composition of your meals is very important. When you combine clean protein, healthy fats, carbs in the form of non-starchy vegetables and whole-grain carbs (in moderation) at your meals, you automatically control the glycemic load of your meals. By keeping the glycemic load low, you avoid raising blood sugar and insulin levels.

Foods that enter your bloodstream quickly (simple carbs) promote weight gain, and food that enters slowly promotes weight loss. The reason is simple—if you eat 150 calories worth of beans and 150 calories worth of candy—the sugar in the candy enters your bloodstream immediately and any calories you are not using right then are stored as fat. The sugar from the beans is absorbed slowly because of the fiber and protein content and your body has a greater opportunity to burn them rather than store them as fat. The fiber also prevents all the calories from being absorbed.

Eat rhythmic, structured meals, which simply mean scheduling your meals every three to five hours. Get into a rhythm so your body burns the fuel you put into it steadily. Eating regularly keeps your insulin and glucose levels stable and prevents that ravenous hunger that convinces you it is ok to eat whatever you can get your hands on!

I have to mention Intermittent Fasting here again (you can re-read the chapter in Section One on Fasting.) Fasting in general is an extremely healthy practice. This is one of the easiest forms of fasting to start with. You still get to eat each day, and in my experience feel only mildly hungry, if at all. Here's the basic idea: you eat all your meals during the day during an eight hour window (10 am to 6 pm, for example) and don't eat outside of this time period. This gives you a 16-hour fast during a 24-hour period with a very minor adjustment to your normal eating schedule. This also seems to be the best option for women, as extended fasting can actually be counterproductive. Most of your fast is accomplished while you are sleeping so it makes it very easy. After about 12 hours of not eating, your glycogen reserves get tapped out and your body needs a new energy source. The body releases fat cells into the bloodstream, which travel to your liver and are burned for energy. Insulin levels go back down and your metabolic measures improve.

Remember, when you eat, a hormone called Leptin is released, which tells your brain that you are satiated or full, at least for the moment. Your insulin levels should decrease and the cycle starts again the next time you eat.

However, if you eat too often, your insulin levels remain high and you can lose insulin sensitivity (also known as insulin resistance), which can lead to diabetes. This is why I recommend weaning yourself from the snacking habit. People who eat small meals throughout the day often have this issue because they never allow their insulin levels to drop to a naturally low level. High levels of insulin signals your body to go into a fat storage mode instead of a fat burning mode. This is the opposite of what you want.

Eat slowly and mindfully. Don't eat on the run—sit down, set a plate and give thanks to God for what you are eating. Eat slowly and chew thoroughly. Pay attention to the flavors, textures and aromas! Enjoy your meals. If you wolf your food down, your brain doesn't have a chance to register that you ate and were satisfied, and chances are you will be looking for a snack even though you ate enough.

Alkalinity

Strive to keep your body in as alkaline a state as possible. When you are in an acidic state, your body tends to shuttle minerals from your bones and teeth to buffer the acids, and this can lead to osteoporosis, dental problems and mineral deficiencies. It also buffers the acid by moving it into fat tissue, which ends up making it impossible to lose the fat since it is protecting your body from over-acidity!

Regulating your water consumption is the first step to alkalizing. Drinking green drinks and eating green vegetables are extremely alkalizing. Making sure to get adequate minerals is also important. Including the Himalayan crystal or sea salt will be alkalizing and will add minerals to your diet.

BUMP UP: Include quality green foods like spirulina, chlorella, Kamut and Moringa and use one every day to stay alkaline. The bonus is that green foods such as these are such nutrient powerhouses; they can safely replace a multi-vitamin and provide all the vitamins, minerals and other nutrients in a wonderful, easy to absorb whole food form!

Here's a pH drink recipe I came across that you can include occasionally: to the juice of one lemon, add ½ teaspoon of baking soda and let it foam up. Once it stops, add 12-16 ounces of water and sip to alkalize your system. I would suggest sipping through a straw so as not to harm your tooth enamel.

You can also take a warm bath to which one cup of baking soda and one cup of Magnesium flakes or Epsom salts have been added to alkalize and relax your body.

Spices

Include a variety of spices and herbs in your meals. They will not only add flavor and interest, but they boost the nutrient value and even help you burn fat, cut appetite and reduce inflammation. For example, curcumin, a compound in turmeric, when combined with piperine (a compound in black pepper), has been found to inhibit growth of stem cells that fuel breast cancer! One-half teaspoon of cinnamon daily balances blood sugar, lowers cholesterol and suppresses appetite! Here are some specific ones to include and why:

- ✓ **Basil:** This herb that perks up Italian food is anti-inflammatory, reduces water retention and bloating, and functions as an adaptogen (a substance that helps your body adapt to stress), as well as reducing fat buildup in your liver while detoxifying your body.
- ✓ **Black Pepper:** It is known to help the body burn more calories through the process of thermogenesis, its piperine content helps your body absorb nutrients more efficiently and is thought to interfere with the formation of new fat cells. A new study even revealed that black pepper could help fight against obesity by reducing body fat and blood sugar levels.
- ✓ **Cardamom:** This spice helps lower blood sugar and regulate insulin which helps suppress your appetite.

- ✓ **Turmeric:** Inflammation is the root of all disease and is believed to also be a root cause of weight gain and obesity. Turmeric is anti-inflammatory and an antioxidant, and some studies have shown it prevents the growth of fat tissue. Taking turmeric with black pepper may boost its bioavailability up to 2000%.
- ✓ **Hot Peppers:** The capsaicin in cayenne and chili peppers stimulates your brain to release feel-good brain chemicals, boosts thermogenesis (fat burning), reduces belly fat and suppresses appetite.
- ✓ **Cinnamon:** A half-teaspoon of Ceylon cinnamon stabilizes blood sugar levels and improves insulin sensitivity, is anti-inflammatory, is an excellent fat-burning spice and even helps reduce belly fat accumulation.
- ✓ **Cloves and Coriander:** Both boost metabolism and increase weight loss.
- ✓ **Cumin:** This anti-inflammatory spice is a great fat burner that also aids in digestion. One teaspoon can help you burn up to three times more body fat!
- ✓ **Garlic:** It contains phytochemicals that break down fat deposits, may prevent formation of fat cells and helps with metabolism of fats and carbs.
- ✓ **Ginger:** It is known to reduce appetite and reduce cravings and can boost your metabolism by about 20% for three hours.
- ✓ **Mustard:** This is another metabolism booster. One teaspoon of spicy or whole-grain mustard increased metabolism by up to 25% for several hours after eating. According to another study, eating ¾ teaspoon of powdered mustard seeds a day burns an extra 45 calories an hour. I put powdered mustard seed in my scrambled eggs and whole-grain spicy or siracha mustard on my burgers.
- ✓ **Parsley:** It can reduce blood sugar levels which can help control your appetite and make the processing of food into energy more efficient.

BUMP UP: Use some black pepper with other herbs and spices to increase your body's ability to absorb the nutrients they contain, increase nutritional value and block fat production. Put cinnamon in your cup of tea. Chinese Five Spice Powder combines cinnamon, nutmeg, allspice, cloves and black pepper—a virtual powerhouse! Black pepper will boost bioavailability of anything it is paired with, so I even put some in my green tea to get more benefit from its many nutrients.

Teas

Another way to get more herbs is to drink a variety or combination of teas. You can combine several to create your own flavor blends: Tulsi lemon/ginger and hibiscus; Kombucha green and oolong; peppermint and Tulsi; fenugreek and hyssop; blueberry and lemon; black chai and yerba mate; valerian and chamomile—use your imagination! You can also include fresh herbs like rosemary, cilantro and basil.

I make my morning tea a powerhouse by combining black chai or green chai with oolong, yerba mate, matcha and hibiscus teas with cinnamon, cloves, ground fennel, black pepper, cardamom and ginger. I steep and blend in my blender with a tablespoon of pasture butter, a tablespoon of MCT oil and a scoop of collagen. You'll find the recipe on my website in the Recipes section under My Morning Tea.

Starchy Vegetables and Friendly Grains

Eat starchy vegetables and whole grains **in moderation**. I can't stress that enough. If you choose to add them, pay close attention to how they affect you and whether your weight begins creeping up. You can easily structure your meals with just healthy fats, protein, lots of non-starchy veggies and only include the starchy veggies or grains occasionally – maybe only on the weekend. You need carbs – it's never healthy to eliminate an entire macronutrient. However, non-starchy veggies are the best source of carbs.

BUMP UP: If you include whole-grain pasta or even rice or quinoa, combine them with a lot of veggies and a half cup of beans. Include more veggies than actual pasta or grain and add some balsamic vinegar to your tomato sauce – it lowers the glycemic index and adds a ton of flavor.

Be sure to properly prepare your whole grains by soaking them. It's easy— the night before simply cover the grain (oats, quinoa, millet, brown rice— whatever) with a combination of one tablespoon plain yogurt, kefir, Amasai, apple cider vinegar or one teaspoon sea salt and enough water to cover. Cover and leave on the counter overnight. When ready to prepare the next day, simply drain and cook in fresh water or stock as you normally would. The harmful phytates are deactivated and all the nutrients are released for your body to use easily.

You will still create your nutrient-dense, fresh, whole food meals around the basic ingredients from the lists in weeks three and four.

Here's how a sample meal plan for a week might look. The meals average between 1200 and 1500 calories. While I don't focus on calories, I find it makes it easier for people who use an app like "My Fitness Pal" to be able to track what they are doing. The sample meals do not include snacks as that's one of the goals in restructuring how you eat. Recipes that follow are marked with an asterisk:

Day One (approx. 1200 calories)

Breakfast: mushroom/two egg omelet using two teaspoons coconut oil; one slice whole grain or gluten free bread spread with one teaspoon coconut oil or pasture butter; tea

Lunch: Green salad (as much as you like) with raw vegetables of choice (peppers, celery, carrots, cucumbers) dressed with one tablespoon flax or olive oil and raw apple cider vinegar and topped with leftover baked, sliced chicken or turkey

Dinner: Tuna (one can chunk white) with 1/3 cup chick peas, 10 ounces spinach*

Day Two (approx. 1400 calories)

Breakfast: one or two hard-boiled eggs; protein shake* (make it cherry today); tea

Lunch: can of sardines (or substitute four ounces of any fish you prefer) in olive oil, drained, topped with two tablespoons salsa on one slice whole-grain, gluten free or sprouted toast or one whole-grain or gluten free wrap

Dinner: four ounces baked chicken, roasted broccoli*, baked sweet potato with one tablespoon flax, olive oil or butter, salt and cinnamon (have the potato if no starchy carbs at breakfast or lunch)

Day Three (approx. 1240 calories)

Breakfast: scrambled eggs with red & green peppers and scallions, one slice whole-grain bread with two teaspoons coconut or flax oil; tea

Lunch: four ounces chicken-mushroom burger*, romaine lettuce salad with cucumbers, olives, capers and tomatoes, dressed with one tablespoon hemp oil and balsamic vinegar; tea if desired

Dinner: four ounces baked fish (salmon, flounder, cod—whatever you like) seasoned with lemon-pepper; steamed green beans and roasted tomatoes with two teaspoons flax or olive oil

Day Four (approx. 1200 calories)

Breakfast: one cup plain, whole milk, organic Greek yogurt mixed with stevia, vanilla extract and cinnamon or half a bottle of plain kefir or Amasai, over fresh berries; one high protein muffin*; tea

Lunch: Turkey-spinach burger*, mixed raw vegetables (baby carrots, sliced red and yellow peppers)

Dinner: Chef Salad with romaine lettuce, tomatoes, one avocado sliced, dressed with one tablespoon flax or olive oil and fresh lemon juice and topped with two sliced, hard-boiled Omega-3 or cage free eggs

Day Five (approx. 1250 calories)

Breakfast: spinach-tomato-dill two-egg omelet; **or** ½ cup soaked old-fashioned or steel cut oats with stevia and cinnamon, allspice and nutmeg and two tablespoons chopped walnuts; tea

Lunch: one cup lentil soup* with ½ cup cooked buckwheat* (if no oats at breakfast) or one package Miracle Noodles*

Dinner: mushroom-zucchini chicken burger* and grilled zucchini and eggplant

Day Six (approx. 1450 calories)

Breakfast: blueberry-banana protein shake*; two hard-boiled eggs; tea

Lunch: ½ cup brown rice, 1/3 cup beans (kidney, chick peas, black beans—your choice) and ratatouille

Dinner: one roasted turkey thigh, leftover grilled vegetables from Day Five

Day Seven (approx. 1275 calories)

Breakfast: two sunny-side up, soft boiled or poached eggs, one slice whole-grain, gluten free or sprouted toast spread with two teaspoons pasture butter or ghee; tea

Lunch: leftover brown rice, beans and vegetables from yesterday

Dinner: almond crusted chicken fingers*, green salad with vegetables of your choice dressed with one tablespoon flax, hemp or olive oil and apple cider or balsamic vinegar

The plan allows for two servings of fruit per day, and you can certainly either use a fruit in your smoothie or include it with a meal. As I have said earlier, I encourage you to begin to eliminate snacking between meals. If you find yourself looking for something, try a cup of tea or bone broth or drink another glass of water. Often we are really thirsty, not hungry.

If you truly find you do better with a small snack between meals, here are some suggestions.

Snack suggestions:

- ✓ one serving of fruit (apple, pear, peach, nectarine, plum) or one cup melon chunks or berries and ¼ cup nuts; fruit is approximately 75 calories, and nuts are about 200 calories with 8 grams protein. Tahini (mix two teaspoons lemon juice to one tablespoon organic, unsalted tahini and combine) with raw vegetables or 13 Mary's Gone Crackers original crackers
- ✓ Tahini and 13 crackers: 230 calories, 5 grams protein.
- ✓ Avocado (one) with lemon—(drizzle juice over sliced avocado) 322 calories, 4 grams protein.
- ✓ 25 Kalamata olives – 100 calories, 2 grams fat, 6 grams healthy fat.
- ✓ Apple slices with nut butter (two tablespoons peanut, cashew, walnut, almond, sunflower seed butter spread on one sliced, organic apple) 300 calories, or one tablespoon nut butter spread into two or three stalks of celery, 120 calories.
- ✓ Raw vegetables (baby carrots, sliced peppers, celery, cucumbers)—0 calories—with three tablespoons tahini (270 calories) or hummus, approximately 100 calories.
- ✓ 70 calorie whole-wheat pita bread with two tablespoons hummus (approximately 200 calories).
- ✓ One cup plain Greek yogurt, a few drops liquid stevia, vanilla and one serving of fruit.
- ✓ One bottle any flavor Beyond Organic Suero Viv or Kombucha.
- ✓ One ounce dark chocolate (at least 70-80% cacao or higher).
- ✓ Two Greek Yogurt Deviled Eggs* (116 calories, 11 grams fat, 3 grams carbs).

✓ Four or five cups air-popped popcorn (150 calories or less). For a special treat, lightly spray with spray olive oil and dust with Braggs Nutritional Yeast Seasoning. You will be licking your fingers! This is a grain, so use this one only occasionally.

Treat Days:

Once you have reached this point, you can schedule a planned "treat" day once a week. (Some plans refer to this as a "cheat" day. Let's not consider it "cheating" since you are sticking to the plan 80-90% of the time.) We never want to create negative emotions like shame and guilt. Remember you can eat whatever you want to, just not every day. So enjoy your "treat" days, you earned them!

Periodically take a day and eat what you want within reason. You can save this for a day when you may be going out to eat or on the weekend. Do not use this as an excuse to pig out or binge! But realize that no food is forbidden! Choose foods you really love and have some as a reward for your consistent efforts. The next day go right back to the plan. I suggest you schedule a treat day once every week or two – but not more often. It's good for the soul and as you'll see below, for your body, too.

Dr. Mercola is a huge fan of the ketogenic diet, and while this plan is not that, something he says relates to what I am telling you here about treat days. He says as beneficial as a ketogenic diet is for your mitochondria, he doesn't recommend staying on it for an extended period. He suggests using a cyclical diet – feast-famine because by increasing carb and protein intake once or twice a week, you increase ketone levels and blood sugar actually drops. The key is after a day or two you go back to the original plan or in his case, the ketogenic diet, which is the fasting stage for the rest of the week.

IF you want to give yourself some extra help during the treat days, particularly if you are having more carbohydrate foods, consider using a carb blocker supplement before those meals. Two I particularly like are listed in the resources. These can be great tools in keeping insulin levels stable when your meal is on the high carb side.

I also suggest that you plan some non-food rewards as you achieve your goals. Buy a new outfit or piece of clothing (in a smaller size?); earrings; get a manicure/pedicure; new haircut/style/color; buy yourself a book, CD or

DVD you've been wanting; schedule a movie night or girls/guys night; be creative and celebrate each step toward your ultimate goal!

Maintenance

Once you have achieved your weight goal, you can adapt the plan a little more. Now you can add a little more whole grain **IF** you choose to. For example, you might have quinoa with breakfast, a slice of whole-grain, gluten free or sprouted bread with your lunch; and a sweet potato with dinner.

However, pay close attention to how the addition of the carbs makes you feel. Do you feel tired, achy, bloated or gassy? Are you gaining weight? Cut back. If a particular carb is to blame—avoid that for a while and reintroduce it at a later time and re-evaluate. You don't have to add in more grains or starchy carbs if you are satisfied, feel well and are easily maintaining your goal weight without them.

You can try carb cycling as well. This cycling strategy can be especially helpful if you reach a plateau.

I explain my method in the last section of alternating your meal plans between the no starchy carb days from weeks one and two, your basic plan from weeks three and up where you eat specific, healthy whole grains and starchy carbs, in moderation and only at breakfast and lunch, and finally a high carb day where you add extra carbs.

Here are two supplements to have on hand for those times you go off— holidays, vacation, parties or just those days we all have. Besides the carb blocker supplements I mentioned above, another supplement you might consider is the herb Gymnema Sylvestre, which is a well-known sugar metabolizer. Particularly if you will be having more sweets (holiday treats, birthday cake?), this may be helpful in limiting the damage sugar can cause. Another that I like is Sweet Eze. (There are links for all products mentioned on the Resources page.) Be sure to run any supplement you try by your doctor to be sure there is no contraindication, especially if you are on any medications.

EXERCISE BUMP UPS: If you needed one more reason to write your exercise session in your daily planner and keep your appointment, exercising five times a week has been shown to reduce levels of C-Reactive protein, a marker for inflammation in the body that is the underlying cause of degenerative disease, by 30%.

So, besides committing to exercising at least three days a week, but preferably five or six, here are some additional tips to bump up your results:

Walking

Walking is considered the simplest form of exercise, important for good health and suitable for all age groups. Benefits of walking include: indirect massage of internal organs, boosting metabolism, relieving stress, improving circulation, promoting clear, effective thinking and as we said in Week Five, it is weight bearing exercise and it strengthens bones.

What makes it a "fitness walk" is the "belly button-to-spine" action — sometimes called a "tummy tuck" — that will make your walk more effective, protect your back and engage your abs.

As you walk, draw your belly button toward your spine. That deep layer of muscle is key to supporting your back. It stabilizes the middle of your body so your legs can move with much more power. It also engages your core, which in turn helps engage other muscle groups as you walk.

As little as 120 minutes of walking per week may reduce mortality risk in older adults. Meeting or exceeding the activity guidelines of 150 minutes of moderate activity per week in the form of walking lowered all-cause mortality by 20%. Walking for six hours or more each week lowered the risk of death from respiratory diseases by 35%; heart disease by 20% and cancer by 9%. Walking 140 to 175 minutes per week added anywhere from three to seven years to an individual's life span!

Vary your routine regularly. Cross-training is a good strategy. If you just walk for one hour on a treadmill set at the same speed and incline every day, very quickly your body will adapt and you will burn fewer calories. At least every two to three weeks (and preferably each time you exercise) vary the length of time, intensity, speed, number of reps and order of exercises. For example, if you walk three miles a day for two weeks and do those three miles in 45 minutes, in week three, walk four miles Monday, two miles Wednesday and three miles Friday, or alternate walking and jogging for interval training. Do something to vary the routine.

Same idea when doing weight training—alternate between body weight exercises like pushups, chair dips, crunches, lunges and squats; dumbbells, exercise bands, kettlebells and medicine ball. Change the position of your hands in the pushups, the number of reps, speed; do different types of squats using different body positions.

Timing

Dr. Mercola says breakfast and exercise are two of your most important health strategies, and I agree. In fact, exercising in the morning has special benefits. According to many studies, the best time for most people to exercise is in the morning for several reasons.

The biggest benefit is that those who schedule their exercise in the morning are most consistent. Getting your exercise done before the urgencies of the day can interfere is a huge benefit. If you wait until later in the day, chances are great that something else will come up and you will skip exercising.

Also, for many of us who begin our days quite early, we are tired by the end of the day and don't have the enthusiasm or energy required to follow through on our plans.

Finally, when you exercise at night you stimulate your system when you are better off relaxing and preparing for a restful night's sleep. Exercising too close to bedtime can cause you to have trouble falling asleep.

A little bonus is this: if you exercise early in the morning, *before* you eat your breakfast (water and even a green drink or cup of coffee or tea is fine), you tend to burn more calories. Just be sure to then eat a healthy, balanced, protein-rich breakfast to nourish your muscles.

BUMP UP: When lifting weights (or doing pushups), try doing your reps very slowly—up to the count of three and lower to starting position to the count of three. Lifting more slowly activates more muscle. Believe me, you will feel the difference. Once you have improved your fitness level, you could consider doing High Intensity Interval Training (HIIT). This can be done with cardio as well as weight training. However, it's best to run this by your doctor and be sure you are ready to take your training to the next level.

Pay attention to the way you feel as you exercise—be mindful. Be aware of tightening your abdominal muscles when doing abdominal work. The muscles respond more when you are concentrating on them. Be aware of how your body responds to what you are doing and visualize the result you want: firmer legs, slimmer hips, or a flatter belly; feel the muscles working. It may sound a bit "out there"—but it's scientifically proven to work.

Practice good posture. Be aware of your posture whether you are sitting or walking. Lift your rib cage, tighten your abs, relax your shoulders and draw them back slightly. Be aware of how good you feel as you walk or sit and periodically thank God for a strong, healthy, pain-free body! (Try sitting on a stability ball or balance disc while working at the computer or watching TV – it will engage your core and help you remain intentionally aware of your posture.)

Get up and move periodically throughout the day. So many of us sit at a desk for at least eight hours a day and we don't realize just how bad all that sitting is for our health. Numerous studies show rates of heart disease, diabetes and obesity are doubled and even tripled in people who sit a lot. A study in the *International Journal of Obesity and Related Metabolic Disorders* found people who sat for long periods daily (7.4 hours or more) were significantly more likely to be overweight or obese than those who reported low daily sitting levels (less than 4.7 hours a day).

Here's why: when you are sitting, the circulation of lipase, an enzyme that absorbs fat, stops. Therefore, instead of being absorbed by your muscles, fat continues to circulate in your bloodstream where it may end up stored as body fat, clogging arteries or otherwise contributing to disease. Simply standing up instead of sitting engages muscles and helps your body process fat and cholesterol more efficiently, regardless of the amount of exercise you do.

ScienceDaily.com confirms this: the enzymes in blood vessels of muscles that are responsible for 'fat burning' (lipase) are shut off within hours of not standing. In fact, after just one hour of sitting the production of fat burning enzymes declines by as much as 90%! Periodically standing and moving turns those enzymes back on. Since people are awake 16 hours a day, when they sit much of that time they lose the benefit of increasing metabolism throughout the day.

This is part of the reason I suggest doing some body weight exercises on your bathroom breaks at the office! Your body can only tolerate being in one position for about 20 minutes before it starts to feel uncomfortable, according to the Mayo Clinic. So about every 15 minutes, stand, stretch, walk around or change your position for at least 30 seconds. Stand up while you talk on the phone or while watching TV and take frequent "intentional exertion" breaks! If you need to – set a timer to remind you to get up and move every 30 or 40 minutes!

The average person can burn 60 extra calories each hour just by standing instead of sitting. Over the course of a day, this can add up to a lot of beneficial health effects.

So get up—frequently—and move that magnificent body God gave you!

Secrets that Increase the Benefits of Your Fitness Routine

1. You can boost your calorie burn by 50 calories each time when you slow down, practice good posture and good form. You call on fewer muscles and burn fewer calories when you do cardio while slouching over rather than standing tall with good spinal alignment. Good posture also allows you to take in more oxygen so besides your workout feeling easier, you burn more calories as well. Research also shows that standing to do strength training slowly boosts calorie burn by about 50 calories per 30 minute session. It may not sound like much, but it adds up over time!

2. The importance of drinking enough water is clear. Since nearly every cell in the body is composed of water, they don't function efficiently without it during exercise, according to experts at California State University in Fullerton. Without adequate hydration, you'll tire more quickly and your workout will feel more difficult than it should. Recent studies found dehydrated people did three to five fewer repetitions per set while strength training. While it's important to be well hydrated before and during exercise, it's also important to replace what is lost through sweating and heavy breathing.

3. A survey finds that listening to music while you exercise increases the duration and intensity of your cardio session. Researchers discovered that runners who listened to motivational rock or pop music exercised up to 15% longer—and felt better doing it. The reason for this benefit is that the music helps you focus on intensity.

4. It is important to choose activities you enjoy and will do consistently. If you try to do something that you really dislike and dread doing, chances are great that you will begin skipping sessions. Researchers found the top predictor of consistent adherence was choosing an enjoyable form of

exercise. There are so many different things to choose from, there's no excuse to force yourself to do something you hate.

5. Most women neglect strength-training. If you're one of them, it may be the number one reason the number on your scale isn't moving. Strength-training builds muscle, which boosts metabolism. Here's something you may not know: people who combine aerobic and resistance training eat less—517 fewer calories a day—than those who do only cardio, according to a study in the *Journal of Sports Science and Medicine*. Combining both types of workouts may increase satiety hormones, boost the body's ability to break down food and stabilize blood sugar, so you feel full longer, says study author Brandon S. Shaw, Ph.D. This one trick alone can result in losing 12.5 pounds a year.

Endurance or Burst Exercise

Endurance exercises like long-distance running or working on a gym machine for an hour actually break down muscle, stress your immune system, and may even cause weight gain. Now before you ditch the endurance exercises altogether, a long hike or a longer, slower cardio session once in a while is perfectly fine. Personally, I wouldn't rely solely on that type of exercise. To jump-start your body into fat-burning mode and kick up your metabolism, you can try burst training or high-intensity interval training (HIIT). The bonus is when you do this first thing in the morning, it causes an oxygen deficit that your body needs to make up during the day, which will cause greater fat loss.

*Be sure to weigh yourself once each week and keep track of your meals, snacks, water intake and how you feel in your food log DAILY. Even when the seven weeks are over, I hope this has become a way of life for you, so continue to use your food and exercise log – it will keep you on track.

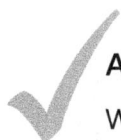

ANN'S PERSONAL TIP: ————————————————

When I can't get out and enjoy a walk on our local trails with my husband or my girlfriend, I often do a workout DVD. My favorites are 20 minute HIIT workouts (links will be in the resources). Sometimes I do a 10 minute kettlebell workout and then just include 20 jump squats in the morning, three or four sets of high knees throughout the day, and 20 jumping jacks at the end of the day. Jumping is a great way to move lymph, and that's important to fight off colds and viruses. You can also use a rebounder or mini trampoline for less impact on your joints. I often use Dr. Mercola's Nitric Oxide Dump exercise. You do it three times during the day waiting at least three hours between each session. It only takes five or six minutes each time, but it is a great workout and a real time saver. It also boosts your immune function. Link is on the resource page.

RECIPES

You can find lots more recipes in the recipes tab on my website.

Ann's Protein Muffins (Gluten Free)

Dry Ingredients:

- ✓ 1 cup gluten free flour—1/2 cup quinoa flour, ¼ cup almond flour and ¼ cup coconut flour
- ✓ (Or any combination you like)
- ✓ ¾ cups quinoa flakes or old fashioned oats
- ✓ 1 scoop whey, collagen or other protein powder
- ✓ 1 cup unsweetened, flaked coconut
- ✓ 4 tsp. aluminum free baking powder
- ✓ 1 tsp. baking soda
- ✓ 4 tbsp. Lakanto, coconut sugar or rapadura (unprocessed sugar)
- ✓ 1 tsp. sea salt
- ✓ ¼ tsp. guar gum or a scoop of organic psyllium husk powder

Wet ingredients:

- ✓ 3 eggs (Omega-3 or cage free)
- ✓ 4 tbsp. olive, avocado or coconut oil
- ✓ 3 mashed bananas or 1 cup unsweetened applesauce*
- ✓ *Can also substitute 1 cup canned pumpkin

Combine wet and dry ingredients until thoroughly combined. You can add in wild blueberries, cranberries, dark chocolate chips, chopped frozen cherries, chia seeds, flax seeds, sesame seeds, pine nuts, walnuts or whatever add-ins you like.

Bake at 350 for 20 minutes for large muffins, 12-15 minutes for mini muffins. Makes 12 large muffins or 16-20 mini muffins. They freeze very well.

Basic Protein Shake

This is my basic protein shake recipe – I just switch up the ingredients to change the flavors. I often use it as a meal replacement for breakfast, lunch or dinner.

For a cherry protein shake:

- ✓ 12-16 oz. water or cooled, brewed tea or cold brewed tea**
- ✓ 1 scoop whey, collagen or other protein powder
- ✓ 1/3 cup frozen cherries (or strawberries, raspberries)
- ✓ Generous handful of organic greens (kale, spinach, chard, romaine lettuce, parsley)
- ✓ 1 small banana, cut up
- ✓ 1 small avocado (optional)
- ✓ Flax, chia, hemp seeds or sunflower or pumpkin seeds
- ✓ 1 small scoop of organic psyllium husk powder
- ✓ 1 teaspoon unmodified potato starch (optional)
- ✓ Ice cubes (optional)
- ✓ Superior Reds powder (optional)

Put half of liquid in blender—add whey and Superior Reds if using—add in fruit, greens, and seeds or nuts. Cover and blend; add in ice cubes, if using, and continue blending till frothy and creamy. I use frozen cherries so I don't need ice cubes.

To make Blueberry-Banana Smoothie, substitute 1/3 cup frozen wild or fresh blueberries and Superior Purples powder;

To make Peach, Pineapple or Mango Smoothie, substitute ½ cup frozen peach slices or mango or pineapple chunks and Superior Oranges powder.

To make chocolate fudge smoothie, use chocolate fudge whey protein and an additional tablespoon of unsweetened, organic cacao. An avocado in this one makes it extra creamy!

**I also alternate what tea blends I use for each. For example, I steep one tea bag each of Yogi Rose Hibiscus Skin Detox tea and Bigelow Cranberry Hibiscus tea for the cherry or any red fruit smoothie.

For the blueberry smoothie, I may steep Bigelow Benefits Blueberry and Aloe herbal tea with Bigelow Wild Blueberry Acai or substitute a bag of Purely Purple tea for either of those.

For the peach, pineapple or mango smoothie, I combine Bigelow Benefits Ginger and Peach or Perfect Peach herbal tea and Bigelow Benefits Chamomile and Lavender herbal tea.

For the chocolate smoothie, one of my favorite combos is Bigelow Benefits Chocolate and Almond herbal tea and Bigelow Jasmine Green tea or Bigelow French Vanilla.

Ann's Oats

- ✓ ½ cup of old fashioned oats or steel cut oats, soaked
- ✓ ¼ cup of oat bran
- ✓ 1 tablespoon plain Greek yogurt, Amasai or kefir
- ✓ Cinnamon, nutmeg, ginger, allspice, cardamom and/or pumpkin or apple pie spice
- ✓ Water
- ✓ Stevia or one or two organic dates*
- ✓ Almond, cashew or coconut milk

Possible add-ins: sesame or other seeds, walnuts, pine nuts, mashed or sliced banana, 1 Tbsp. any nut butter, berries

Soak the oats overnight in 1 tbsp. of either yogurt, Amasai or kefir and enough water to cover. In the morning drain. Bring 1-1/4 cups of fresh water to a boil and add drained oats and oat bran. Stir continuously over medium high heat until you get a creamy consistency. Pour into a bowl with a tight fitting cover and let sit about 5 minutes to absorb all liquid and get creamy. *If using a tablespoon of nut butter—add it now and stir in while oats are very hot so the butter melts and is well incorporated. After it sits a few minutes sprinkle stevia, spices and whatever other add in's you choose and a little almond or coconut milk to make it the consistency you like and enjoy!

*If you want to use the dates as your natural sweetener, I suggest you chop them up and combine them with the oats when you cook them so they have a chance to soften and release their sweetness as they cook.

Chicken Mushroom Burgers

- ✓ 1 lb. ground chicken (Also delicious with grass-fed beef or any other ground meat)
- ✓ 4-5 finely chopped organic baby bella, Shitake or white mushrooms
- ✓ 2-3 Tablespoons cooked, mashed lentils

- ✓ ½ a grated, raw zucchini or 1 grated carrot or finely chopped onion, red bell pepper or shallot
- ✓ Cumin, sea salt, freshly ground black pepper, fennel or whatever seasonings you like

Combine all ingredients - form into 4 good sized patties and either cook in non-stick pan sprayed with a little spray oil or on an oiled grill or under broiler until completely cooked through.

Turkey-Spinach Burgers

- ✓ 1 lb. organic ground turkey (or beef, chicken, veal, bison or lamb)
- ✓ 1/3 of a 10-oz box frozen, chopped, organic spinach, thawed and squeezed dry
- ✓ Seasonings of your choice: sea salt, black pepper, chipotle seasoning, herbs de Provence; basil and oregano, etc.
- ✓ 1/4 cup cooked, mashed lentils or other beans
- ✓ 1 small zucchini, grated

Break up the spinach and add to the turkey along with the beans and season as desired. Divide into 4 patties and cook as above. Can top with a thin slice of Beyond Organic Cheddar or Havarti and allow to melt and serve on a grilled Portobello cap.

You can also make them "Greek" burgers by including some crumbled feta cheese and seasoning with oregano, sea salt, pepper, cinnamon and nutmeg.

Lentil Soup
(I make a big pot—divide it up and freeze in one-serving containers and just thaw in fridge overnight before I want to use it)

- ✓ 4 cups water and 1 cup chicken, vegetable or beef stock (I like Kitchen Basics) or a good quality organic chicken or beef bone broth
- ✓ 1 cup brown lentils
- ✓ 4 stalks celery chopped
- ✓ 2 carrots chopped
- ✓ 1 onion chopped
- ✓ 4 bay leaves

- ✓ 4-5 cloves of garlic—whole
- ✓ Herbs de Provence or basil and oregano
- ✓ 1 tsp. sea salt, fresh ground black pepper
- ✓ Thyme, dill weed
- ✓ Several dashes kelp-type seasoning like Maine Coast Organic Dulse Granules or Sea Kelp Delight Seasoning
- ✓ 1 small 8 oz. can organic tomato sauce

Bring lentils, vegetables, bay leaves, water and stock to a boil on high heat. Reduce to low heat and simmer covered 1 hour until lentils are tender. Add in all seasonings and tomato sauce and continue to simmer an additional 15-20 minutes. Can also add frozen chopped or fresh spinach or kale if desired.

I serve it like my mom used to—put 1 tbsp. extra virgin olive oil and 1 tbsp. raw, organic apple cider vinegar into the bowl and then fill with the soup.

Buckwheat

- ✓ 1 cup buckwheat groats
- ✓ 2 cups water or combination water and stock or bone broth
- ✓ 1 tbsp. yogurt, Amasai, kefir or apple cider vinegar

Overnight, soak buckwheat, covered on counter, in water to cover with 1 tbsp. of yogurt, kefir, Amasai or vinegar

Next morning drain and combine with 2 cups liquid (water and/or stock)—bring to boil, lower heat and simmer covered for 30 minutes.

Can also add chopped, sauteed vegetables or any seasoning that appeals to you if it will be used as a side dish. Add cinnamon, stevia and almond or coconut milk if it's a breakfast dish.

Christopher's Tuna with Spinach and Chick Peas
(My son Chris made this up and I tried it for dinner and loved it—and spinach has been found to help with protein synthesis—a win-win!)

- ✓ 1 can of solid white tuna in water or canned wild salmon

- ✓ 10 oz. box frozen, organic chopped spinach, thawed and squeezed dry
- ✓ ½ cup of any beans you like (I especially love chick peas)
- ✓ Mrs. Dash Lemon pepper seasoning
- ✓ 1 tbsp. olive or avocado oil
- ✓ Combine all ingredients and heat gently in a pan—can be eaten warm or at room temp.

Creamy Green Tuna Salad

- ✓ 1 can solid white tuna
- ✓ ¼ of a medium onion chopped finely
- ✓ 1 stalk of celery chopped finely
- ✓ 1 avocado mashed
- ✓ Juice of ½ lemon
- ✓ Chili lime spice or Mrs. Dash Lemon-Pepper seasoning

Break up tuna in dish; add mashed avocado, lemon juice, onion, celery and seasoning and combine well.

Serve on lettuce or in one whole grain or gluten free wrap.

Ratatouille

- ✓ Zucchini, eggplant, one onion, 4 ribs celery, 1 bulb fennel chopped, Brussels sprouts, carrots (or whatever vegetables you prefer)
- ✓ 1 can organic, fire roasted diced tomatoes
- ✓ Sea salt, black pepper, cumin, turmeric

Using 2-3 tbsp. olive or avocado oil heat a large nonstick pan; chop vegetables and add to pan, season and add can of tomatoes and half can of water. Bring to boil and then lower to simmer, cover and cook 30-45 minutes until veggies are tender.

Almond-Crusted Chicken Tenders
Makes 4 servings

- ✓ Cooking oil spray

- ✓ ½ cup almond "flour" which is simply ground almonds
- ✓ ¼ cup whole-wheat, spelt or brown rice or oat flour if you are gluten free
- ✓ 1 ½ teaspoons paprika
- ✓ ½ teaspoon garlic powder or granulated garlic
- ✓ ¼ teaspoon sea salt
- ✓ ¼ teaspoon freshly ground black pepper
- ✓ 1 ½ teaspoons avocado or olive oil
- ✓ 2 whole eggs beaten
- ✓ 1 pound chicken tenders (you can substitute boneless, skinless thighs if you prefer dark meat, as I do)

1. Preheat oven to 450°F. Line a baking sheet with foil. Set a wire rack on the baking sheet and coat it with cooking spray.

2. Place almond meal, flour, paprika, garlic powder, salt and pepper in a food processor and mix thoroughly; with the motor running, drizzle in oil; process until combined. Transfer the mixture to a shallow dish.

3. Whisk eggs in a second dish. Add chicken and turn to coat. Transfer each piece to the almond mixture; turn to coat evenly. (Discard any remaining egg and almond mixture.) Place the chicken on the prepared rack and coat with cooking spray; turn and spray the other side.

4. Bake the chicken until golden brown, crispy and no longer pink in the center, 20 to 25 minutes for tenders, a little longer for thighs.

Baked Chicken Thighs

- ✓ 2 skinless, boneless free range, organic chicken thighs (works great with turkey thighs too – only cook longer as they are not usually boneless, are much larger and remove skin if not free range and organic)
- ✓ Coconut Aminos (about ¼ cup)
- ✓ Juice of one lemon
- ✓ Cumin, Herbamare and black pepper, paprika

Put thighs in baking dish, add liquid Aminos, lemon juice and season. Add enough water to the pan to keep liquids from burning. Sprinkle with paprika for color. Bake at 350 degrees uncovered for about 25 minutes. Tender, juicy and delicious!

Lamb Chops Greek Style

- ✓ 4 lamb chops
- ✓ 2 garlic cloves, finely chopped
- ✓ Sea salt, ground black pepper, dried mint leaves or finely chopped fresh mint leaves
- ✓ 1 tablespoon olive oil, 2 tablespoons fresh lemon juice
- ✓ Combine garlic, seasonings, oil and lemon juice in a ziplock bag.

Add lamb to bag; seal and shake to completely coat lamb in marinade.

Allow to marinate for at least 15 minutes, up to an hour.

Heat another tablespoon of oil in pan over medium high heat and cook lamb 3- 5 minutes on each side for medium-rare. Serve and enjoy!

Liz's Easy, Perfect Salmon

My daughter seems to have perfected this recipe, originally found on Pinterest - so I'm sharing her version which comes out perfectly cooked (not overcooked which ruins salmon) and just delicious.

- ✓ Preheat a pan on medium heat.
- ✓ Season your wild caught salmon with sea salt and pepper on both sides.
- ✓ Heat 1 tablespoon of avocado or coconut oil - just enough to coat the bottom of the pan.
- ✓ Put your salmon filet in skin side up. Shake the pan a bit to be sure it didn't stick. Cover the pan and cook until the filet is white about halfway through (depending on thickness - 6-8 minutes).
- ✓ Flip the filet, squeeze about 2 tablespoons of lemon juice over it. Cover the pan and turn the heat off. Let the fish continue cooking and steaming in the covered pan until cooked to medium (about 5-8 minutes).

Roasted Sweet Potatoes or Vegetables

- ✓ Peel and cut sweet potatoes (or any potatoes) or vegetables (cauliflower, broccoli, asparagus, squash) into 1-2" chunks
- ✓ Put on cookie sheet, drizzle with 1-2 tbsp. of avocado oil

- ✓ Season with sea salt, cracked black pepper and whatever spices you like

Roast at 350-375 degrees for 30 minutes or until lightly brown and tender. I especially love cinnamon, salt and black pepper on sweet potatoes!

My Favorite Chili

- ✓ 1 Tablespoon olive or avocado oil
- ✓ 1 large onion, diced
- ✓ 1 shallot diced
- ✓ 4 cloves of garlic, chopped finely
- ✓ 4 organic carrots scrubbed and diced
- ✓ 1 red bell pepper diced
- ✓ 2 chipotle in adobo sauce, chopped finely and 2 tablespoons of the sauce included
- ✓ 1 teaspoon to 1 tablespoon Saveur chili spice (depending on the level of spice you like)
- ✓ 1 15.5 oz. can each black beans and red kidney beans, rinsed well and drained
- ✓ 2 lbs. grass fed and finished, organic ground beef or bison (you can substitute ground chicken or turkey if you prefer)
- ✓ 1 28 oz. can organic crushed tomatoes or tomato sauce
- ✓ 1 16 oz. can organic, fire roasted diced tomatoes
- ✓ Granulated garlic, sea salt, cumin, black pepper (I held back a bit on the chili powder because I don't know how spicy people will want it – but season it to your taste)

Saute onion, shallot and garlic in 1 teaspoon of the oil until softened, about 4 minutes. Season with salt and pepper. Remove to crockpot.

Sautee carrots and bell pepper in remaining 2 tsp. oil, salt and pepper until softened. Remove to crockpot.

Brown meat in pan with a little oil or spray with spray oil to prevent sticking and season with salt and pepper. Remove to crockpot.

Add the beans and tomatoes and season with spices. Cover and cook on low for at least 2 hours or more. It tastes better the more you heat and reheat!

Baked Fish Filets

- ✓ 1 lb. fish filets like cod or flounder or any other mild white, flaky fish
- ✓ ½ cup organic salsa*

Spray a baking dish lightly with spray oil. Put filets side by side in dish. Pour salsa over.

Cover with aluminum foil and bake at 350 degrees for approximately 15 minutes or until fish is cooked through and flaky. Serves 2.

*If your salsa is very liquid you may want to put the fish on a rack in the pan that's been sprayed with spray oil first and then top with the salsa so the excess liquid falls to the bottom and your fish isn't too wet.

Breakfast (or Lunch) Quinoa

- ✓ ½ cup of quinoa, rinsed and soaked in water to cover overnight with a tablespoon of yogurt or Amasai
- ✓ 1 cup water (if breakfast meal) or stock or bone broth if lunch
- ✓ Seasonings – cinnamon, allspice, nutmeg for breakfast, stevia to taste;
- ✓ Cumin, black pepper and coriander for lunch. If this is a side dish you can also add chopped, lightly sautéed or roasted veggies of your choice

Drain quinoa, bring water or stock to a boil, add drained quinoa and seasonings; if adding cooked veggies you can add now or at the end; lower to simmer, cover and cook 12-15 minutes.

Allow to stand for 5 minutes to absorb all liquid. Fluff with a fork. Season to taste. Makes 2 servings.

Beyond Organic "Ranch" Dressing

- ✓ 1 cup of healthy mayo*
- ✓ 1 bottle of plain Amasai
- ✓ Chopped: chives, parsley, dill, garlic
- ✓ Onion powder, sea salt, pepper

Combine the mayo, herbs and seasonings. Add 1 bottle of plain Amasai and whisk together until smooth. Serve over greens or with anything you normally serve ranch dressing with.

*Spectrum Organic Olive Oil Mayonnaise is good and my preferred choice is Primal Kitchen Avocado mayo.

Besides the nice creaminess, you get the added benefit of healthy fats, which help release more of the nutrients in salad vegetables as well as probiotics and enzymes.

Boosted Bone Broth

Quite often, especially during the cold winter months, I enjoy a big mug of bone broth daily. When I do a fast or modified fast, bone broth is usually an important part of my day. I can't always make a batch from scratch, so using powdered bone broth solves the problem.

There are quite a few high quality bone broth powders you can purchase to make this easier, and I take advantage of this! I like keeping this on hand and then all I have to do is put a heaping scoop in my mug, add some boiling water and enjoy.

I often like to boost my bone broth. I figure why not get the most bang for my nutritional buck?

I often include a scoop of MCT Oil Powder and I always add about a quarter teaspoon of Himalayan Crystal Salt.

Depending on my mood, I enjoy adding different herbs and spices, including:

- ✓ Turmeric
- ✓ Onion Powder
- ✓ Chili Spice
- ✓ Ancho Chili Powder
- ✓ Rosemary
- ✓ Seasoned Salt
- ✓ Sage
- ✓ Coriander
- ✓ Garlic

- ✓ Ginger
- ✓ Curry Powder

You get the idea - the only limit is your imagination and what appeals to you at the moment.

Soaking Nuts and Seeds

Soaking nuts and seeds is not difficult. Luckily the process of soaking is essentially the same for whatever type of nut or seed you chose to prepare, although the timing varies slightly to accommodate for differences in fat composition, size, texture, etc. Traditional soaked nuts and seeds are made by following these basic steps:

1. Measure out 4 cups of raw, unsalted, organic nuts/seeds into a medium sized bowl

2. Cover with filtered water so that nuts are submerged

3. Add 1 tablespoon natural, unrefined salt (Himalayan Crystal or Celtic Sea)

4. Allow to stand covered on the counter for about 7 hours, or overnight

5. Rinse nuts to remove salt residue and spread out in single layer on a rack to dehydrate.

6. Dry in the oven at a low temperature (generally no higher than 150°F) or in dehydrator for 12-24 hours or until nuts are slightly crispy.

These steps are adapted from Nourishing Traditions by Sally Fallon. If you want more information on this and other traditional food topics, I highly recommend getting a copy of her book.

Cauliflower Tots

- ✓ 1 medium head of fresh cauliflower
- ✓ 1/2 small onion diced finely
- ✓ 1/4 cup grated Parmesan Cheese
- ✓ 1/4 cup coconut flour or gluten free bread crumbs
- ✓ 2 large eggs beaten

Preheat the oven to 350 degrees. I covered a large baking sheet with aluminum foil and liberally sprayed it with cooking spray.

Cut cauliflower into florets and add to a large pot of boiling, salted water. Cook until fork tender, about 7 minutes. Drain thoroughly and put into a food processor. Pulse for a few seconds until it breaks down into the size of rice grains. Don't pulse too much or it will go too far and become too mushy to form.

Add the pulsed cauliflower to a large bowl. Stir in the onion, cheese, coconut flour or breadcrumbs and beaten eggs. Mix until thoroughly combined. It should be close to mashed potato consistency.

I used a small ice cream scoop to scoop up some of the mixture and then formed it into a little log (tater tot shape more or less). Place them on the prepared baking sheet about an inch apart. Spray lightly with the spray oil.

Bake for about 20 minutes. Carefully flip them and bake 10-15 more minutes until crisp and golden. Serve with hummus, pesto, salsa or ketchup - whatever dipping sauce you like! Enjoy without guilt!!

Stuffed Portobello Mushrooms

My husband has gone gluten free and after 30+ years of marriage is finally a little more open to trying some different foods and meals. He's always been very picky and very limited in what he thought he liked. I made this and expected him to say he didn't like it but got just the opposite response - he loved it! It's easy to make and very healthy. I urge you to try it - even for your pickiest eater!

- ✓ 1/4 cup teff grain
- ✓ 1 small onion chopped
- ✓ 1 tablespoon oil (coconut, avocado or olive)
- ✓ 1/2 cup stock or bone broth
- ✓ 5 Portobello mushrooms, stems removed and gills scraped out
- ✓ 1 package organic chicken or turkey sausage - cooked and chopped into about 1/4" dice
- ✓ 1/2 cup shredded mozzarella or whatever cheese you like

First I made some teff grain. I cooked 1/4 cup of teff in a little less than 1/2 cup of broth for about 20 minutes. I fluffed it with a fork as soon as it had absorbed all the liquid and set it aside.

Put about 1 tablespoon of oil in a pan and sauté the chopped onion until it is softened and golden - remove from the pan and add in the chopped sausage. Sauté it to heat it through and crisp it up a bit. Combine the teff, sausage and onion together in a bowl.

Put the prepared Portobello caps stem side up on a baking sheet and bake for about 15 minutes at 350 degrees. Pour off the liquid that they release and put them back on the baking sheet. Fill each with the teff/sausage filling, top generously with the shredded cheese and bake another 10-15 minutes at 350 degrees or until the cheese is all melted.

My husband never even asked about the teff - it just melded with the sausage and cheese and gave it a nice filling consistency.

Let me know what you think if you try it!

Salmon Burgers

These salmon cakes are the perfect snack or meal. They have a high quality, clean protein, veggies, healthy fat and fiber! They're quick and easy to make ahead and have ready for the week and are just delicious.

- ✓ 14.75 oz. can of wild Alaska Salmon
- ✓ 1/4 cup coconut flour
- ✓ 2 tablespoons ground flax seeds
- ✓ 1 teaspoon chili powder (I like Ancho)
- ✓ 1 tablespoon of cumin (very anti-inflammatory!)
- ✓ 2 eggs, beaten
- ✓ 2 tablespoons lemon juice
- ✓ 1 small organic zucchini, grated
- ✓ 1 small organic carrot, grated
- ✓ 1 stalk of organic celery, finely chopped
- ✓ Coconut or avocado oil for cooking

Drain the salmon and break up with a fork in a large bowl. Add veggies, seasonings, flax seeds and coconut flour and combine well. Add eggs and lemon juice and mix well. Using a tablespoon, scoop out a generous spoonful and form into small patties. Cook in a small amount of healthy oil 3-4 minutes or until golden over medium heat; gently flip and cook the other side.

You can eat them warm or cold as a high protein snack.

*My very favorite way to serve them is to roast some sweet grape tomatoes with olive or avocado oil, salt, pepper and oregano (I do this often in the summer when I have so many grape tomatoes from my garden) and then combine them with a good quality Kalamata type olive and spoon some over each burger. It's absolutely delicious!

Kale Chips

These are really easy to make and I've done them both ways - using a bunch of organic kale and also using organic baby kale. Using the baby kale results in a much more delicate chip and they burn very quickly - so if you want a crunchier, more substantial chip, a bunch of organic kale is the way to go.

Strip the leaves off the tough, center rib. Tear into healthy bite-sized chips. Preheat the oven to 350 degrees.

Spread your chips out on a baking sheet lined with either parchment paper, foil or a
silicone mat.

Either lightly drizzle them with avocado oil or lightly spray with spray olive or avocado oil.

Season them any way that appeals to you. My daughter's favorite seasoning is chili-lime spice. I've used Herbamare, granulated garlic, and sea salt and black pepper. They are delicious, too. Use whatever appeals to you.

Bake for 5 or 10 minutes (depending on your oven) until crisp and crunchy - but keep an eye on them because they will burn quickly.

You can substitute spinach or another leafy green or even Brussels sprouts as well.

Greek Yogurt Deviled Eggs

- ✓ 2 hard-boiled eggs
- ✓ 1 Tablespoons organic, plain yogurt
- ✓ 1 teaspoon mustard
- ✓ Salt, pepper, paprika

Carefully remove the yolks. Mash with the yogurt, mustard, salt and pepper.

Refill the center of the egg whites with the mashed yolks and sprinkle with paprika.

Bone Broth from Scratch

Be sure the bones are from organic, grass-fed beef or organic, free range chickens or turkeys.

1. Place bones into a large stock pot or crockpot.

2. Add two tablespoons of apple cider vinegar (I use Braggs) to water prior to cooking. This helps to pull out important nutrients from the bones.

3. Fill pot with filtered water to just cover bones. Leave plenty of room for water to boil. Adding beneficial herbs like turmeric, ginger, black peppercorns, rosemary, parsley and even cinnamon helps leverage all the great healing power of your bone broth and enhances the potency (and the taste) of your broth. I also include one organic onion cut in quarters (unpeeled), one or two organic carrots, scrubbed, unpeeled and cut in thirds, one or two ribs or organic celery and a head of organic garlic broken into cloves, each clove crushed to release the allicin. You don't need to peel the garlic as you will remove it. You can also include an unpeeled knob of whole ginger if you like.

4. Heat slowly. Bring to a boil and then reduce heat to simmer for at least 6 hours. I typically leave beef bone broth simmering for 24 hours.

5. Cook long and slow. Chicken bones can cook for 6-48 hours. Beef bones can cook for 12-72 hours. A long and slow cook time is necessary in order to fully extract the nutrients in and around the bones.

Strain out the veggies and bones and discard. I do scoop out the marrow from the beef bones and add it back into my broth. I then add back some fresh chopped veggies and simmer another 30-45 minutes until the vegetables are tender and then it's done! After cooking and straining, the broth will cool and a layer of fat will harden on top. This layer protects the broth beneath. You can discard this layer but I include it. You can also skim it and use it in cooking. It's delicious.

Refrigerate if you plan to be eating it that week or freeze for later use. Sip on the broth or use as the base in a nutrient-dense soup.

To make a chicken bone broth use:

4 lbs. organic, free-range chicken wings, necks and feet (ask the butcher for these!) and the veggies and herbs from above or whatever you like. Don't forget to include the apple cider vinegar.

The procedure is the same. Cook long and slow. Chicken bones can cook for 6-48 hours. When it finishes cooking, strain the solids out of the liquid and allow to cool, cover and refrigerate. Use it within one week or freeze.

It makes a delicious base for my Immune Boosting Probiotic Soup. You can find the recipe on my website in the Recipes tab.

Bone broth contains collagen to make your skin supple and radiant. But that's not all! Other valuable nutrients include gelatin, hyaluronic acid, chondroitin sulfate, proline, glycine, calcium, phosphorus, magnesium and potassium. When you drink a broth made with a good source of red marrow, you are drinking all those stem cell factors that ultimately build your body's strength and support your own immune function. However, that's why you need to know that the bones are truly from humanely raised animals that are grass-fed and finished to get the best quality nutritional value.

This delicious, mineral-rich broth can be used to make soup to support smooth, strong skin and reduce cellulite. While that's certainly a plus, that isn't why I made it. It is also excellent for healthy joints, bones, ligaments, tendons, and gums, which is why I wanted to make it. It is an amazing healing food and provides the body with raw materials to rebuild stronger and healthier cells. I'm all for that! So when I do my periodic three-day fast, I just add a serving of bone broth each day and I have to say it is delicious and very satisfying as well.

The high quality marrow these beef bones contained (which I scooped out into my broth) is excellent for building blood, if you have anemia, and boosting immune function. The gelatin in bone broth protects and heals the mucosal lining of the digestive tract and helps aid in the digestion of nutrients. AND the amino acid glycine in the broth is a potent liver detoxifier. Perfect addition to detox days.

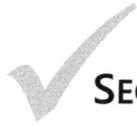

SECTION THREE
INTEGRATING SPIRIT AND SOUL

Weeks One and Two: Spirit & Soul Detox

I combine spirit and soul because they overlap although they are distinct and different. While your spirit is the core of who you are and the realm of God-consciousness, your soul is your mind or intellect, will and emotions – your personality and what makes you uniquely you – which receives information from both your spirit and your physical five senses. Your soul is where you think, feel and make choices.

When we talk about your spiritual heart (not the blood pump in your chest), it receives information from both your spirit and your soul. Your brain receives input from your physical body as well as from your soul. Essentially, your soul is the conduit for your spirit and your body. Your heart is a combination of your spirit and your soul. It's important to also realize that just as your physical body has five senses – sight, taste, smell, touch and hearing – so does your spirit!

We are told in Romans 8:6 NKJV: *"For to be carnally minded is death, but to be spiritually minded is life and peace."*

As you can see, they are all interrelated and each one impacts the other areas. You are an integrated tri-part being. You are a spirit, you have a soul and you live in a physical body. Therefore, you can't just detox or nourish your physical body and be truly healthy and whole in the best, fullest sense of that word.

Here in the US we have an obesity epidemic. Too many of us weigh more than we should, or want to. There are thousands of diets out there because it's not healthy to go through life with a heavy body. Neither is it healthy to go through life with a heavy spirit. Things like offense, bitterness, negativity, worry, selfishness, frustration, pride, hopelessness, and fear make your spirit heavy.

Jesus invites us to *"Come to Me all you who are weary and heavy laden, and I'll give you rest. Take My yoke upon you, learn from Me, for I am gentle and humble in heart and you shall find rest for your souls because My yoke is easy and My load is light."* Matthew 11:29-30

I **love** how the Passion Translation says it: *"Simply join your life with mine. Learn my ways and you'll discover that I'm gentle, humble, easy to please. You will find refreshment and rest in me. For all that I require of you will be pleasant and easy to bear."*

You could say this is His spiritual "diet." While it is simple and elegant, it is not always easy for us to do. However, it is doable and that's why I want to share some thoughts about how you can release the spiritual weights you are carrying around and become light hearted!

Be Sure You are Sowing the Right Seeds

When you plant seeds or plants in your garden, you only reap what you have sown. I typically plant tomatoes, cucumbers, peppers, zucchini and eggplant. Those are the vegetables I reap. I never go to my garden and find green beans on my zucchini plant or broccoli on my tomato plant. It is the same in your body. You can't sow junk food and diet soda and reap a strong, vibrant, healthy body. Seed reproduces after its own kind. You also can't sow bitterness, anger and fear and reap love, peace and joy. I urge you to always keep in mind what you are sowing so you won't be surprised by the harvest you reap.

Why Detox Your Spirit

Because we live in such a toxic environment, this key is first and of great importance. When my computer's fan became clogged with dust, periodically the computer would overheat and just shut down. If your car's filters are dirty and clogged, it backfires, sputters and stalls. When you are clogged with toxins, the same thing happens to you! A clogged digestive filter may result in constipation or indigestion; a clogged respiratory filter may cause chest congestion or asthma; clogged emotional filters may cause depression or anxiety; clogged spiritual filters can result in fearfulness or pride. Just as our autos and computers need periodic maintenance, our spirits, souls and bodies do also in order to keep them functioning well.

How Can You Detox Your Spirit?

Everything begins with the spirit because that is "who" you really are. A clogged spirit will affect every other area of your life. I love to look at scriptures in different versions because each brings out a different nuance.

Proverbs 18:14 explains why spirit must always be first. Let's look at it first in the Amplified: *The strong spirit of a man sustains him in bodily pain or trouble, but a weak and broken spirit who can raise up or bear?* New Century Version says it this way: *The human spirit can endure a sick body, but who can bear it if the spirit is crushed?* The Passion Translation says: *The will to live sustains you when you're sick, but depression crushes courage and leaves you unable to cope.*

How do your spirit and soul become weak, broken or crushed? Unfulfilled expectations, disappointments, frustration and criticism are all possibilities. Perhaps cherished dreams didn't come true or something you worked on so hard to achieve, failed. Maybe you grew up with a significant authority figure in your life (parent, grandparent, teacher, coach) constantly criticizing you, putting you down or telling you, even in subtle ways, that you just were not good enough. That can crush and weaken your spirit. Perhaps you internalized those negative messages and now you are continually beating yourself up, telling yourself you are not smart, or good, or successful, or attractive. Often, without even realizing it, we just pick up where the critical one in our lives left off and continue the same abusive dialogue.

You may continually read scriptures about God's love, but you cannot seem to receive that love because in your spirit and/or your soul you feel unworthy. These negative messages create toxins such as fear, offense, anger, worry, bitterness, resentment, depression, envy and pride, which can then manifest themselves in your life as sinful behaviors. It isn't hard to understand how these toxins could then spill out of you and contaminate your relationships, is it?

Jesus, in speaking to the religious teachers of His day, rebuked them because they were so focused on appearances. He said, "*Hypocrites! You are so careful to clean the outside of the cup and the dish, but inside you are filthy—full of greed and self-indulgence. Blind Pharisees! First wash the inside of the cup, and then the outside will become clean, too.*" (Matthew 23:25- 26 NLT)

The First John 1:9 Strategy

The Bible provides us with a simple, very clear-cut process to begin this detoxification process. I call it the First John 1:9 Strategy. That scripture says:

"If we confess our sins, He is faithful and just to forgive us our sins and to cleanse us from all unrighteousness." I've broken it down into three steps:

- ✓ Acknowledge
- ✓ Agree
- ✓ About-face

Those toxins are sins. Romans 14:23 says whatever is not of faith is sin and I think we can agree pride, bitterness, resentment, fear, worry, anger are not born of faith. So the first step in cleansing your spirit of these toxins is to confess or **acknowledge them to God**. Honestly admit that you are afraid or angry or prideful or anxious—whatever it is. There is really no point in pretending otherwise. God is not surprised by your admission—He already knew about it. This step is for you.

Next, you **must agree with God** that they are sins. Don't make excuses or rationalize. Don't call it a fault, flaw, weakness or shortcoming. Call it what God says it is—a sin. Period. First John 1:10 says: *"If we say that we have not sinned, we make Him a liar and His word is not in us."* That is a very serious allegation.

The last step is to **do a total about-face**—repent! That word means to change your mind or direction completely; move to a higher level. The word repent comes from the same root as penthouse. Rather than rationalizing why certain people "make" you angry or a specific situation "makes" you feel afraid, commit yourself to detoxing that—acknowledge it, agree it is sin and change it. It doesn't serve your highest and best interests. Make a quality decision to completely change your mind about it. Do an about-face. Rise above it. Think ahead of time about the specific situations or people who trigger that sinful behavior or reaction. Decide ahead of time how you will respond differently. You may have to avoid certain situations or people, or decide you will simply refuse to respond at all. God will show you the best way.

One of the reasons this plan is so effective is that it addresses spirit, soul (mind-will-emotions) and body. By now you should be realizing how your thoughts, beliefs and emotions can affect not only your mood but your physical health as well.

You've heard the saying, "you are what you eat." That's true. You may also have heard the saying, "garbage in, garbage out" referring to programming a computer. That's also true. Just as eating toxic, fake "food" will determine your overall health and physical energy, filling your mind and spirit with negative thoughts and beliefs will determine the condition of not only your mood and attitude, but your physical body as well.

Once again, you are totally in control of the type of fuel you choose to put into your spirit, soul and body! Negative emotions increase levels of stress hormones like cortisol. Toxic thoughts can change gene expression as much as exposure to toxic pesticides in your food.

Negative emotions that are toxic include guilt, shame, anger, anxiety and fear. Fear weakens your adrenal glands and kidneys. Sadness not only suppresses effective functioning of your lungs and large intestine, but actually destroys healthy bacteria and digestive enzymes your body naturally makes. Guilt and shame depress the function of your pancreas and stomach.

Some of the most effective "detox" strategies are: being quick to listen, slow to speak and slow to become angry (James 1:19), what I call the 1John 1:9 strategy above; applying the 3 C's (coming up in the Soul Detox section) to detox destructive thinking patterns; being willing to forgive quickly and completely; and being quick to apologize. Clear emotional clutter and just as in housekeeping—stay on top of it. EFT is great for this. Don't allow those toxins to accumulate—determine to keep your "house" swept and clean.

I realize this is easier said than done. Sometimes even when we deeply desire to forgive and understand the importance, we find ourselves unable to do so. This is why I recommend Christian EFT in addition to the other strategies I have suggested.

The Power of Forgiveness

It has been said refusing to forgive someone is like taking poison and expecting the other person to die! You must realize that you do not forgive for the other person's sake. You do so for your own benefit. If you refuse to forgive someone, you are held in bondage and they have control in your life. We are to be directed and controlled by the Holy Spirit within us (Rom. 8:9). Walking in love and forgiveness keeps our faith "channel" clear. Here are some scriptures on forgiveness: Matthew 6:12-14; 18:35; Luke 7:47; Acts 26:18; Ephesians 4:32; Colossians 3:13.

In its most basic form, to forgive is to send the offense away rather than hold on to it. If you hold on to it, it has mastery over you! I strongly suggest you visit Dr. Jim Richard's website at Impact Ministries where he has some excellent resources to help you with this.

So how do you go about forgiving when someone has hurt or offended you? Here are several things you can do.

Journaling is a great way to work through your feelings. If you regularly journal to God, use part of your prayer time to clearly and specifically express all your feelings about this particular individual or situation. By the way, it doesn't matter if it happened two days ago or twenty years ago—if it is still causing you to harbor feelings of unforgiveness, you must deal with it. Be totally honest with God and say everything about it that you want to. Then ask Him what He would say to you about it. Get quiet and write whatever thoughts or pictures you get. Communion with God Ministries has wonderful resources including Dr. Mark Virkler's book, *4 Keys to Hearing God's Voice,* which will teach you two-way journaling. I have found this to be life-changing.

You can also write a letter directly to the person who hurt you. Imagine you are speaking directly to them and tell them exactly how you feel. However, once you have said everything you need to say, do not mail the letter. Don't even save it! Destroy it and throw it away. As you do this, intentionally release all the anger, resentment, bitterness and hurt, and by faith, forgive that person simply because God calls you to. Don't worry if you don't "feel" like you have forgiven them—do it by faith, in obedience to His Word and the feelings will follow.

This is where spirit and soul overlap quite a bit and also where biblically based, Christian EFT is very effective in releasing these emotions that no longer serve you. I will talk in more detail about that.

Visualization exercises are very effective because they access your subconscious mind. This is the part of you that is programmed by your past experiences to react automatically. Even though many of these issues are subconscious and you may not even be aware of them, they can still be affecting you. Every memory is stored in some cell of your body and whenever the right trigger appears, you react without realizing why.

By imagining a different result, you begin to reprogram your subconscious. Imagining the new result while using EFT (tapping) is even more effective and powerful.

God gave us a holy imagination and most of us persist in using it to worry instead of to visualize and imagine things as we wish them to be, which is what God does. Scripture tells us God calls things that be not as though they are (Romans 4:17). That is visualization at its best. First take several deep, slow breaths. Pay attention to your breath and heartbeat and allow your mind and body to become relaxed. Try to imagine the person who has hurt you being attached to you by a big, heavy, black chain. Try as you might, you struggle and pull, but you cannot move away from them. Then you simply ask Jesus to help you. He immediately stands between the two of you and severs the chain. It falls off both of you. You are now free to move wherever you like. You look back to see Jesus has put His arm around the other person's shoulders and walks away with him or her. Now He is free to deal with him or her. Forgiveness frees you and puts the person who offended you into His hands.

Begin to honestly acknowledge any areas that are hindering your spiritual growth and your relationship with God as well as with your family and friends. Where do you need to apply the First John 1:9 Strategy? Do you need to forgive someone? Do you need to forgive yourself? So often we are harder on ourselves than anyone else.

Try the exercises above and begin your spiritual detoxification. You will feel as if a hundred pound weight has been lifted from your shoulders!

Most people in America are overweight. A quick Google search reveals thousands of diets, because it's not healthy to go through life with a heavy body. However, as I said at the beginning of this chapter, it is just as unhealthy to go through life with a heavy spirit. Thankfully, we never have to carry our burdens all alone. If we can entrust them to our Lord just as a small child trusts a parent to help him or her, that spiritual weight will evaporate. Trust me, getting healthier is MUCH easier when you are not dragging a heavy spirit around with you!

What Is Soul Detox

Your soul includes your mind, will and emotions—and so this would include negative, destructive thoughts, speech, habits, attitudes, limiting beliefs, emotions and relationships. 3John 2 says: *"Beloved I wish above all things that you prosper and be in health, even as your soul prospers."* God's will is for us to be healthy and prosper—spirit, soul and body. Negative emotions are toxic to you physically and can affect hormones, digestion and immune function, making you more vulnerable to disease.

Mind: We all fall victim to "stinkin thinkin:" toxic, negative thought patterns that have been created, resulting in low self-esteem, inability to trust, always expecting the worst. How do you know if this is a problem? Listen to your self-talk—are thoughts like "nothing ever goes right for me" or "I'm not good/smart/young/rich/talented enough" your constant companions? These can also be called limiting beliefs. By taking these thoughts captive (2 Cor. 10:5) and renewing your mind to God's Word (Phil. 4:8 and Rom. 12:2)—you are doing what doctors refer to as cognitive behavioral therapy!

I Call It The 3C's - Capture, Cancel and Confess:

This is absolutely critical because your thoughts are words that contain pictures, and every thought produces an emotion. After only six to ten seconds, your thought begins to take root and produces chemicals and hormones that affect your physical body.

The first step is to **capture the wrong thought**. That's what 'taking it captive' means. Be aware and acknowledge immediately that the thought is contrary to the truth of God's Word. Agree right then and there that it is toxic to you.

Now to **cancel that thought**, simply say out loud, "No, I cancel this thought." It's important to say it out loud because you cannot think one thing and say another. Once you speak, your mind must stop and listen. So you truly cancel the thought.

The last step**, confess**, **is the renewing your mind part**. You replace that toxic thought with a God thought. For example, let's say the thought comes to you that you cannot do something. "I can't do this, it's too hard." First capture it—immediately acknowledge the thought—be aware of it. Agree it is contrary to God's Word. Cancel it - say, out loud, "No, I cancel that thought." Then replace it with a God thought. Say, "Of course I can do this. I can do all things through Christ Who empowers me." You must "say" it— hearing yourself is very powerful. Remember the woman with the issue of blood? She thought about Jesus healing others, and then she *continually said, "If I touch the hem of his garment, I will be whole"* (Matthew 9:20). The speech center of your brain controls every nerve in your body!

Now, just repeat that sequence until...until when? Until the pattern is broken and replaced. It is a process and it may take many times of doing this for the same thought until you gain the victory, but if you don't give up, you will win. Through faith and patience we inherit the promises!

You can exponentially accelerate the process if you do the 3C's while tapping.

According to Dr. Caroline Leaf, thoughts have a physical structure and influence the production of bio-chemicals in our bodies. Thinking determines how you function spiritually, emotionally, mentally and physically. Every thought has a corresponding electrochemical reaction. Depending on the type of thought, specific bio-chemicals are released in response.

Happiness, gratitude and love release certain chemicals and sadness, anger and fear release different ones. Thoughts have the power to change your whole system. (As a man thinks so is he! Proverbs 23:7).

Will: According to Dr. Caroline Leaf, it takes at least 21 days to rewire neural pathways and begin building a new thought. Then it takes two more 21-day cycles for a total of 63 days to truly establish a new thought or a new habit.

Regarding negative or destructive thoughts and habits, Colossians 3:5-8 tells us we are to put them off and some translations say put them to death. Whatever you starve—dies! For example, let's use complaining. I suggest you go on a "fast" giving up that particular habit. You have to be vigilant and stop and correct yourself every time you realize you've slipped back into the habit. It takes time, effort and patience, but it can be done. In order to make real changes to your lifestyle, you've got to learn how to change your brain!

The first time you do anything new, a new pathway is created in your brain. The next time you do it, your brain searches to see if you have done it this way before. If you have, it'll follow the same pathway. The more often you repeat that experience or think that thought, the stronger that neural pathway holding that thought or behavior becomes. This is how a thought or action becomes a habit.

Zig Ziglar says: "Motivation gets you going and habit gets you there." It's critical to form the right habits! Consistency is the key!

By repeating a pattern, you strengthen the neural pathways used for this behavior. Repetition creates new pathways in your brain and creates the new habit over time. Every time you deny yourself something (fast), or you repeat a new pattern, your will is involved.

Emotions: If you are holding on to grudges, worry, anger, sadness, bitterness, hurts, disappointments—you must release them. Negative emotions like anger increase levels of cortisol, the stress hormone. Fear weakens adrenal glands and kidneys; sadness suppresses lung and large intestine function; guilt and shame depress digestive function of the stomach and pancreas. Medicine now acknowledges that back pain can be caused by suppressed emotions. (You may not be able to identify these suppressed emotions which become destructive cellular memories, and I recommend EFT for that.)

Forgiveness is critical here—even if the person who has hurt you doesn't apologize—you can forgive them—which is releasing them into God's hands and allowing Him to deal with them as I mentioned before. Forgive yourself! In Philippians 4:6-7 we are given three steps by which we can release these toxic emotions—those keys are: prayer (communing with God), petition (specific, definite requests) and thanksgiving! Then we are free to receive His peace that passes understanding!

The other side of this forgiveness coin is to cultivate the ability to genuinely apologize. Like forgiveness, true apology is an act of surrender. It clears the toxins of guilt, shame and blame and allows you to move forward as you take responsibility for your actions. Guilt is an extremely powerful emotion, much like shame, anxiety and fear. All of these emotions poison you, mentally, emotionally and physically. Guilt and shame stem from feeling you are not worthy or that you are a disappointment—to your parents, yourself, even to God. So a critical step here is to understand and accept the fact that God loves you totally and unconditionally.

I suggest you take some time and meditate on these scriptures and prayerfully journal about your feelings:

John 16:27: *For the Father Himself tenderly loves you because you have loved Me (Jesus) and have believed that I came out from the Father.*

John 17:23: *I in them and You in Me, all being perfected into one so that the world will know You sent Me and will understand that* **You love them as much as You love Me.** This is Jesus speaking!!

Please don't gloss over those words—God the Father loves you just as much as He loves Jesus! That was a life transforming revelation for me. Perhaps reading it in The Passion Translation will help you see this more clearly: *"You live fully in me and now I live fully in them so that they will experience perfect unity, and the world will be convinced that you have sent me,* **for they will see that you love each one of them with the same passionate love that you have for me.** "Wow!

Gratitude is a very powerful, positive force. Matthew 15:36 and 1 Thessalonians 5:18 clearly tell us we are to give thanks *in* all things. Notice it doesn't say we must give thanks *for* all things. There's a difference. Studies have revealed that thankful people:

- ✓ Handle stress better;
- ✓ Are more optimistic;
- ✓ Are more alert and energetic;
- ✓ Attract gratitude and kindness from others; and
- ✓ Enjoy better overall health.

Each day find three things to sincerely thank God for and either write them in your journal in the evening or talk to God about them as you drift off to sleep. Alternatively, you can begin your prayer time in the morning by thanking God for them -- a positive and powerful way to begin any day.

Spend some time and see where you need to deal with some "stinkin thinkin" patterns. Are there some habits you need to replace? What about your emotions? Where do you need to release toxic emotional responses?

These may take some time to change—more than just a week or two. For most of us this is an on-going, continual process. That's OK. Be patient and gentle with yourself, but also be honest. The only way to rid yourself of these spirit and soul "weights" is to honestly acknowledge them and then consistently take the steps necessary to change them.

I want to take a moment to touch on your thinking as it relates specifically to losing weight and getting fit. You may have been overweight most of your life and feel it's a losing battle and you'll never be able to lose the weight. That's a negative attitude toxin you must flush out of your soul! You must begin thinking like a healthy, lean, fit person. There's a saying you may be familiar with—"act as if."

That simply means to act as if what you desire is already true. It's a scriptural principle:

Reportedly, Blaise Pascal told those struggling with their faith to act as though they believed. Pascal believed that even something as basic as acting as though they believed would count as the mustard seed of faith that Jesus promised would remove mountains. Satan hates it when we express faith but loves to hear us express doubt.

So make a commitment today to stop making Satan's day by thinking and saying those negative things about yourself! Act as if you are a lean, healthy, fit person. You will be amazed at how that shift in attitude affects your behavior! You will find it easier to make healthier choices and then you will begin to see progress very quickly and more effortlessly than you may have thought possible.

Quieting the Inner Voice

It's critical that we find ways to quiet the constant inner conversation we all have going on in our heads and change it from negative to positive in order to create vibrant wholeness and true health. We are told in 2 Corinthians 10:5 to *"cast down arguments and every high thing that exalts itself against the knowledge of God, bringing every thought into captivity to the obedience of Christ."*

We covered detoxing or cleansing spirit and soul, including several strategies, like the 3 C's, for taking your thoughts captive and making them line up with the Word of God. Your thinking is critical to health in every area. This is foundational if you are to live in peace (shalom-wholeness).

Meditation has been proven to quiet the mind, relax the body, reduce stress hormones, boost the immune system, lower blood pressure, improve concentration and sleep, relieve headaches and even lower the risk of heart disease and cancer. We are encouraged numerous times in scripture to intentionally fill our minds with God's Word. For example:

- ✓ Philippians 4:8 (Message Bible): *"Summing it all up, friends, I'd say you'll do best by filling your minds and meditating on things true, noble, reputable, authentic, compelling, gracious—the best, not the worst; the beautiful, not the ugly; things to praise, not things to curse."*
- ✓ Joshua 1:8 NIV: *"Do not let this Book of the Law depart from your mouth; meditate on it day and night, so that you may be careful to do everything written in it. Then you will be prosperous and successful."*
- ✓ Isaiah 26:3 NLT: *"You will keep in perfect peace, all who trust in you, all whose thoughts are fixed on you!"*

What I want to suggest here is that in "rebooting" you begin changing how you see yourself and begin meditating on the results you expect to achieve. When those "arguments" flood your mind like "Just eat one cookie—it won't hurt" or "You know you can't lose weight"—cast them down and replace them! If you keep "meditating" on the lies, no matter how much effort you put into it, you will fail! So, if you have a vision board, put a picture of yourself as you used to be and would like to look again. Use your imagination—take a picture of an outfit you have but can't fit into right now and put that in if your goal is to wear it again. Include whatever specifically encourages you.

Next I suggest you write out a few faith confessions to go with that—you should've come up with these when you were setting your goals at the beginning, so go ahead and include them. Need some suggestions? Besides the ones I already suggested, how about:

- ✓ I break every generational curse coming against reaching my healthiest weight right now in the Name of Jesus!
- ✓ I am releasing this weight for the glory of God!
- ✓ I take authority over food addiction right now in Jesus' Name!
- ✓ My body is the temple of God, and I commit to getting it fit for work in His kingdom!
- ✓ Right now I want to make (or learn to make) healthy choices and I can.
- ✓ I only want to put high quality fuel into my body.
- ✓ Right now I want to be able to (or learn to) control my appetite and make good choices easily.
- ✓ I want my body to be firm and toned and to have energy and strength.
- ✓ I enjoy being physically active every day.
- ✓ I want to live (or learn how to live) a balanced life.
- ✓ I want to glorify God in my body.

*Remember to word your confessions in a way you can believe now.
This is why I have suggested adjustments to how you might word these.

- ✓ Then give your vision a title sentence that you can speak to yourself every time one of those negative thoughts settles in your mind like,
- ✓ "I am a vibrant, fit and healthy person."
- ✓ "I glorify God in my body."
- ✓ "I am energetic and fit and I look great."

Pick a statement in the present tense and every time one of those lies or excuses comes into your mind—use the 3 C's to capture, cancel it and confess the truth in its place—and then meditate on the truth—repeat your faith confession to yourself—look at the vision. In fact, do that every morning and evening as well as any time those negative thoughts bombard your mind. You will experience success so much more quickly!

Christian EFT

Jesus not only wants to heal you, He also wants to make you whole. He cares deeply about every detail of your life, about your thoughts, feelings and emotions. He wants to bring you peace and comfort. All you have to do is turn to Him and receive His love and let Him bring healing to your heart and restoration to your soul. Simple, right? Unfortunately too many of us have tried over and over to do just that and seem to be stuck in those negative emotions, thoughts and beliefs even though we believe He is our Healer and wants to heal us. But He doesn't just want us healed of whatever the affliction is, He wants to restore us to wholeness, shalom, peace.

The scripture in 3 John 2 in the Amplified says: *"Beloved, I pray that you may prosper in every way and [that your body] may keep well, even as [I know] your soul keeps well and prospers."*

Since scripture makes a clear distinction between spirit and soul (1 Thessalonians 5:23), I see in this verse that your soul (mind-will-emotional) health is critical to spiritual and physical health and that is what EFT is so effective in addressing.

This is what led me to Christian EFT, and I would just like to give you a simple explanation of what EFT is and how Christian EFT is different. If you are interested in learning more or trying it, you can visit my website and click on the Tapping into Health tab.

First of all, EFT stands for Emotional Freedom Techniques. It is referred to as tapping because we tap on different meridian end points on the face and upper body. I mentioned every memory is stored in the cells of our bodies on a subconscious level. We may have long forgotten an upsetting memory but even though we don't readily recall it, when something happens today that triggers the same feelings, we relive the memory even if consciously we don't recall it.

What EFT does so beautifully is to pull out the emotional charge around a memory and neutralize it. Once you have done that, it no longer triggers the same emotions when a similar conversation or event happens in the present day. What we all crave is peace and quiet and calmness. We want someone to show us how to slow down in life, shut off our fears and anxieties. EFT does all of this and brings us into a closer relationship with our Lord. Second Corinthians 12:9 tells us Christ is our sufficiency. Tapping can teach you to actually live out that verse!

Christian or Biblically-based EFT differs in that we rely on the Holy Spirit to guide us as memories and emotions surface, and we use scripture throughout the process.

You may be wondering what this has to do with weight loss. Your digestive system is very sensitive to your emotions. Healthy emotions lead to healthy choices. Every thought you have has a corresponding emotion, so as Dr. Leaf so eloquently says, you are not only what you eat, but what you think as well!

It's easy to see how negative emotions can lead to emotional eating. It isn't the stress itself but your perception of it that can be so destructive. We all have stress in our lives and it isn't inherently bad. It depends on how we perceive and react to it. Studies have been conducted that showed if the participants believed the stressful thought or event was negative and harmful, it increased their risk of death by over 40%. The participants who didn't perceive it as being harmful actually decreased their risk of prematurely dying. You can change your perception and your body's response to the stress.

https://www.ncbi.nlm.nih.gov/pubmed/22201278

http://psycnet.apa.org/record/2011-30116-001

Often what Christians who are unfamiliar with this energy-oriented healing and self-help technique are a little put off by is that you focus on the negative emotion and memory. We are taught to think and speak what we want to see – not the problem. But in this instance, we must begin by focusing on the negative in order to address and neutralize it.

I was reading a devotional by Joseph Prince about Jesus' restoration of Peter after he had denied him three times. He related Peter thought that with his betrayal and Jesus' death, everything was probably over for him. So he went back to his old job as a fisherman. And that's where Jesus found him, fishing on the Sea of Galilee. The Bible tells us that Jesus gave Peter and the fishermen with him an abundant catch, and also cooked breakfast for them on a fire of coals. You can read the entire account in John 21:1–18. Reliving that scene of men sitting around a fire to keep warm in the early morning must have painfully reminded Peter of what he had done just a few days earlier (John 18:17–18, 25–26). It must have powerfully impacted his emotions and memories.

What was the Lord doing? He was showing Peter that He didn't hold that sin against him, and that Peter didn't have to be afraid of that memory anymore! It struck me that this sounded like EFT in action. Jesus created a clear sensory picture of the painful memory in order to help Peter release it so it would never have the same impact or emotional charge again.

In a nutshell, that is what Christian EFT seeks to help us do. It is extremely helpful in dealing with food cravings and emotional eating.

Weeks Three & Four (And Beyond):
Nourish/Fuel Your Spirit and Soul

Spirit Fuel

Your spirit will not stay strong, vibrant and healthy on one meal a week any more than your body will! Your body requires good, whole physical food and your spirit requires good spiritual food. Here are some excellent forms of spiritual fuel:

Pray and commune with God—make it a daily habit, the first thing you do and what you do all throughout the day.

A daily devotional is also "good fuel." I receive several daily devotionals in my email each morning. Some of my favorites are Word of the Day, God is Doing a New Thing, Sapphires, and Today's Word with Joel and Victoria Osteen. (Links will be on the resource page.)

I always choose a different devotional book to use in my prayer time in the morning. There are many excellent ones out there, so you can choose one that appeals to you. Two that I have especially enjoyed and found spiritually nourishing are *Journey Through the Bible* by Ivey Rorie and *Book of Mysteries* by Jonathan Cahn.

Listen to uplifting praise and worship music. There are so many wonderful CDs. Depending on the style of music you prefer, the choices are endless.

I have come to enjoy listening to Wholetones, which are musical frequencies and tones believed to have been played by King David himself to heal and soothe King Saul in his time of depression. It is therapeutic music played in VA hospitals for veterans. Doctors have found the tones had positive effects on anxiety, pain, mood, and quality of life. Personally, I enjoy playing them in the morning when I am praying and reading my devotional. It just amplifies the nutritional benefit to my spirit! The link to learn more about them is on the Resources page.

Feast on God's Word. As I already said, daily devotionals are one way. You could also read the corresponding chapter of Proverbs for each day of the month using a different translation each month! There are wonderful one-year Bibles that have a specific reading for each day that enable you to read through your Bible in a year. Whichever way you choose to do it, take time to read and study the Bible.

Make your time in the car or cleaning your house a time of spiritual nourishment by listening to teaching tapes/CDs.

Meditate on the Word. That simply means to roll a scripture over and over in your mind. There are several ways to do this. You can take a scripture from your devotions or daily Bible study and think about it: picture yourself in the verse; ask yourself how you can make it part of your life. You can also memorize one scripture a week and as you are memorizing it, think about it, picture it, imagine it and chew on what it would look like in your life. That's what meditation is.

I also highly recommend two-way journaling as I mentioned before. I regularly journal to God in my quiet devotional time and ask Him questions. I have learned to more clearly hear His answers to me, which I then journal. It has truly revolutionized my quiet time. I highly recommend *4 Keys to Hearing God's Voice* by Mark and Patti Virkler.

"Complete" Hydration

Psalm 1:3 (AMP) "And he shall be like a tree firmly planted [and tended] by the streams of water, ready to bring forth its fruit in its season; its leaf also shall not fade or wither; and everything he does shall prosper [and come to maturity]."

As I was praying and thinking about being dehydrated and what the effect is on the body, the Lord showed me something in a way I'd not looked at it before. I work with people so often who are chronically dehydrated that my focus is very much on the physical. However, He showed me that like the woman at the well in John chapter 4, He wanted to get my focus off just the physical to see what is truly important – the spiritual. This is where it all originates and it is the only part that endures, so it's what really matters.

There are several scriptures that talk about the importance of hydration, including the one above. Just as a drought will affect the very root system of trees and plants, it will affect ours as well! When a tree is well hydrated and has a healthy, strong root system, it will withstand the storms that come against it.

If it has been through a long period of drought and its root system has been compromised, you will likely see it totally uprooted after a storm. We are no different. We will either be able to bend and spring back under the pressures of daily life if we are well hydrated or break under the pressure of the storm – and it won't take much!

I talk often about dehydration and how it affects our physical bodies, but I saw clearly what a very small (albeit important) part of it this is. Spiritual dehydration is something we often overlook. We've all experienced feeling our prayers and communion with God are dry. That comes from us – we are not quenching our spiritual thirst with the Living water of the Word. Our spirit becomes parched and withers.

Then there's soul dehydration. We can have a dryness in our thinking, and when things get dry they get brittle and are easily broken. Our thinking, which is part of our soul, can become inflexible.

When our emotions are parched, we get stuck, fatigued – everything seems too hard. We're easily irritated, short-tempered. We snap. We can't properly process our emotions and see the truth. We get stuck in the negative. It's like walking through molasses. It is impossible to properly process our emotions when we are dehydrated physically. Healthy emotions rely on a properly hydrated soul and body.

When our will is parched, we can't make a decision. Either we don't have a clue as to what to do or we just default to whatever seems right or feels good at that moment, even if we know it is not the best choice. It's easy, takes no thought and no self-control. Our will becomes dry, old, brittle and tired, so we avoid exercising it!

We need complete hydration because each of these areas impacts the others. Physical dehydration makes it difficult to properly process emotions and hinders all our bodily functions. Spiritual dehydration sucks the joy from our lives. Mental dehydration is exhausting. Emotional dehydration is paralyzing. When our will is parched and starved for moisture, we are imprisoned, trapped and unable to make progress.

Dryness speaks of lifelessness. Be mindful of staying completely hydrated.

Soul Fuel

Remember your soul includes your mind, will and emotions and it is very critical to nourish each with the right fuel. If you feed your mind with negative, angry, resentful, bitter, fearful thoughts, you will then begin to feel those same emotions. Your will becomes weak. Who wants to create healthier habits when their mind is full of anxiety and fear and their emotions are going haywire? No one!

I want to speak a little here about how your emotions and your words affect your digestion and nutrition. It is critical to know what state of mind you are in *while* you eat. When you are angry, stressed or fearful, those emotions cause biochemical changes in your body that directly and negatively affect your digestion. Proverbs 17:1 says it's better to eat a dry crust with peace and quiet than a house full of feasting with strife! That is literally true for the health of your body and the efficiency of your digestion. You don't digest food properly or effectively if you eat when you are angry or upset.

Proverbs 17:22 says a cheerful heart is good medicine. We don't usually take verses like these literally; however, I believe God included them because that is exactly what we need to do. Scientific research and studies have proven that positive, happy thoughts activate the parasympathetic nervous system which rebuilds, heals and nourishes the body by stimulating your immune and digestive systems.

Not only does stress affect the physiological function of the gut, but it has also been shown to actually cause changes in the composition of the microbiota, your good bacteria.

Dr. Masaru Emoto did fascinating scientific research on how water responds to words—spoken or written. He chose to study water because it is the most abundant substance on earth and in our bodies as well. He found and dramatically illustrated that words of love, blessing and gratitude created perfect, beautiful, ordered ice crystals, and words of anger, fear or hatred created ugly, distorted ones. This gives new meaning to the power of prayer to sanctify our food! You can see pictures of his research online.

So, approach your meals in a positive, peaceful, grateful state of mind and it will make a huge difference.

Feed your mind healthy, positive fuel which will nourish your emotions and strengthen your will:

- ✓ Read motivational, inspirational books; watch uplifting TV shows, movies, DVDs.
- ✓ Listen to uplifting, soothing music—whatever your favorite is. In 1Samuel 16:23, King Saul found relief when David played the harp for him. Recent studies confirm that listening to music you love can lower blood pressure, reduce stress and improve your health. In fact, music bypasses the conscious mind and is a potent stress reliever.
- ✓ Enjoy and appreciate nature, art, music, literature, a perfectly ripe piece of fresh fruit, a favorite meal.
- ✓ Pamper yourself—take time out and do something you enjoy. Read, take a walk, paint, color, write, dance, sing, crochet, play a sport, sit and daydream! Many of us feel guilty simply enjoying life, but Ecclesiastes 8:15 clearly tells us He created life for us to enjoy!
- ✓ Nourish and fuel yourself, peacefully, mindfully and carefully every single day!

WEEK FIVE:
SPIRIT & SOUL EXERCISE

Spirit Exercise

The fruit of the spirit are your "spiritual muscles," and they must be exercised daily to stay fit! Some of the same strategies in nourishing the spirit are also good for exercising it! Prayer, worship, praise, reading, studying and meditating on the Word are excellent exercise. In addition, memorizing scripture and speaking faith confessions are also spirit-builders.

Be a "doer" of the Word by sowing good seed daily! Seed is so much more than just finances. Here is a list of some seed you can sow:

Thoughts, words, money, kindness, love, respect, faith, honesty, peace, discipline, integrity, prayer, patience, encouragement, compassion, understanding, generosity, excellence, grace, mercy, forgiveness, joy, obedience, enthusiasm, ideas, expectation, dreams, gratitude, liberty, praise, worship, consistency, talents, gifts, sincerity, a smile, truth, faithfulness, loyalty, action, perseverance and tenacity.

Keep your spiritual muscles firm and strong by using them every day.

You Have the Final Word

Our personal decision in every situation is the difference between victory and defeat. On one side of us is the world's "wisdom," and on the other side is the wisdom of God. It's an old fashioned tug of war, but who determines how it all turns out? We do! Each one of us is what Kenneth Copeland calls "the establishing witness."

How things look, what's happened in the past, what our friends or family say are all things that we allow to become evidence. You know what I mean. Your family says, "You aren't overweight, just pleasantly plump, and you have such a pretty face. You don't need to lose weight" or "You're getting too thin—you look sick" or "Have a piece of cake, what could it hurt? You're getting to be a health fanatic."

You may think—maybe they're right! Why am I putting the effort into something I'll probably end up failing at anyway? If that's the mental tug of war going on in your mind, STOP IT NOW!! Instead, what does the Word say about whatever you are trying to accomplish? What does God say about you?

Get in agreement with God's Word. It isn't difficult. Just pray according to the Word and establish your witness. Once you do your part in this equation, then God does His: He confirms His Word. He says you can do all things through Christ Who strengthens you; He tells you to choose life; that He is your Healer and that you are already healed; He says you have the mind of Christ and that you are a winner, an overcomer, the head and not the tail, more than a conqueror!

What does this have to do with exercise? Replace those negative, failure beliefs with what God says about you. You have the final word—you're the deciding witness. Exercise your authority. Speak up!

Soul Exercise

Mind: Exercising your mind is as easy as learning something new. It can be anything! A new skill: knitting; crocheting; painting; drawing, sketching, doing cross-stitch; writing; cooking; playing an instrument; dancing; singing; martial arts; a different type of exercise like Pilates or tai chi; learn a new language; do puzzles; word searches; scrap-booking—the list is endless. Allow your curiosity free reign.

Will: The very same thing that detoxes your will strengthens and exercises it as well! Do a voluntary fast. A fast doesn't just have to involve food. You can fast from criticizing, complaining, reading the newspaper, drinking soda or watching TV news—once again, it can be anything. Any time you commit to do (or not do) something *and* you keep your word, it is like doing a weight lifting session for your will!

Emotions: One of the best ways to exercise positive emotions is to practice refocusing events. Choose to see any person, situation or circumstance from God's perspective rather than simply from a human point of view. By changing how you see something, you change your perception of it, which determines your emotions toward it. Our perception is our reality.

Refocusing

Refocusing, as I call it, is finding the positive in any situation. There is always something we can learn and some positive we can glean from it. We can't always control what happens to us; however, we ALWAYS have the power to choose to control our response to it. Making that conscious decision to challenge thoughts, not just accept them, begins with renewing your mind to the Word of God.

The apostle Paul illustrated this concept beautifully for us in 2 Corinthians 4:8 NLT: *"We are pressed on every side by troubles, but we are not crushed. We are perplexed, but not driven to despair. We are hunted down, but never abandoned by God. We get knocked down, but we are not destroyed."* Talk about finding the positive!

You can choose to be a victim or a victor who intentionally makes a decision to learn from events and move on. Things can be catastrophes or challenges; obstacles or opportunities; stumbling blocks or stepping stones. People can be stubborn, shy and slow or determined, sensitive and thorough. We are told in 1 Corinthians 13:7 Amplified: *"Love...is ever ready to believe the best of every person..."* That includes thinking well of yourself!

Instead of dwelling on the negatives, refocus your lens and find the hidden blessing! You can do this with nearly every situation—even the most traumatic ones. This may sound simplistic, but by choosing to practice this Biblical principle, you will dramatically reduce your stress level and improve your health and relationships as well. Just remember that this is a process. Don't be hard on yourself as you learn to refocus. Changing any habit takes time, and this is no exception.

It is also very important to acknowledge and deal with your emotions honestly. If you try to repress emotions, you may be able to hide them for a time, but sooner or later they will erupt! Repressed emotions are always inappropriately expressed. And, they NEVER just disappear. I suggest you speak the truth in love and allow yourself to fully feel your emotions—both positive and negative. You may find that using Christian EFT to first neutralize the negative emotion and then to "tap in" God's truth is not only effective and powerful, but extremely refreshing as well.

Week Six:
Spirit & Soul Rest and Reboot

Spirit Rest & Reboot

I mentioned earlier that the spirit and soul overlap, and the place they overlap is what we refer to as the heart – not our physical heart – but our spiritual heart. That spiritual heart is just as essential to your physical health as your physical heart. People talk about dying from a "broken heart" and this is not just a poetic way of saying they were sad. It has been scientifically proven to be true.

Studies have shown that the loss of a loved one raises your own risk of sudden death, known as the "bereavement effect."

Broken heart syndrome (stress cardiomyopathy) is a real medical condition, triggered by acute, major stress or shock, such as the death of a loved one. In fact, the emotional stress of losing a loved one through divorce, death or any other circumstance can have as powerful of an impact as full-blown depression. Heartbreak can have a devastating impact on your emotional health and the loss of a vital connection can lead to the literal breakdown of the physical functions of the heart.

- ✓ Proverbs 14:30 NASB says: *"A tranquil heart is life to the body..."*
- ✓ The New King James says: *"A sound heart is life to the body..."*
- ✓ The Amplified says: *"A calm and undisturbed mind and heart are the life and health of the body..."*

What is a "sound, calm, undisturbed and tranquil" heart that is life to the body?

I read that the Hebrew word for "sound" is the same root word that is translated as "heal" in other verses. Joseph Prince explains that: The root word for Rapha means to "relax." The pictographs from this word are: a head, a mouth, and grace. So, "The head and the mouth speak of grace."

This is why it is so important to have a peaceful, relaxed heart if you want to truly be healthy and whole. It may seem impossible not to get stressed out, depressed or worried, but 1 Peter 5:7 AMPC tells us: *"Casting the whole of your care [all your anxieties, all your worries, all your concerns, once and for all] on Him, for He cares for you affectionately and cares about you watchfully."*

So learning how to bring rest and refreshing to your heart will bring life and health to your physical body.

Sabbath rest allows you to realign and reflect on the goodness of God. It allows you the time to concentrate fully on Him and allow Him to be present to you in a powerful way. By the way—you can make any day a day of Sabbath rest! God tells us to come away and spend time with Him. If He rested on the seventh day, we certainly can use one day a week to allow Him to refresh and restore us spiritually as well as physically. (I even take a "Sabbath day of rest" from my supplements and let one out of every seven days be supplement free.)

Use that time to pray, read scripture, watch a Christian movie or teaching on DVD, listen to praise and worship music, meditate on one of God's qualities—His faithfulness, gentleness, goodness, mercy or grace. The point is to spend time with Him and allow Him to speak to your spirit.

Soul Rest & Reboot

Mind: There are all different types of Christian relaxation tapes you can listen to that will help you clear and relax your mind. Impact Ministries and also Dave Martin Ministries have some excellent meditation CDs you may want to try.

I also mentioned I love listening to the Wholetones CDs. They are seven songs recorded in seven unique frequencies that are healing and soothing. They also have a set of Wholetones lullabies as well to encourage peaceful sleep. I have and love both.

Will: Learn to delegate! It sounds simple but for some of us it can be difficult. Delegate means to let it go—let someone else do it! You can delegate chores, responsibilities and even worries or problems. Simply do as scripture tells us and "delegate" them to the Lord by casting that care upon Him (1Peter 5:7), leaving it in His hands and then moving on. Easier said than done—but doable! God wouldn't tell us to do it if we couldn't. Remember, it's a process—you may have to cast and re-cast that care each time the thought of it comes to you. Just keep putting it back into His hands and you'll find you have to do it less and less frequently. Practice makes progress.

I provided a link to my Worry Journal Exercise on the Resources page.

Emotions: We tend to either relive the past or yearn for the future and we miss the gift of today! This is "the present" and it is God's gift to us. God described Himself as "I AM." Young's Literal Translation renders it: 'I AM THAT WHICH I AM" In Charity Kayembe's wonderful book, Everyday Angels, she says: "With the Lord one day is as a thousand years, and a thousand years is as one day. (2 Peter 3:8) God is I AM - not I was or I will be - so we want to be present and live into His eternal now."

All too often we find ourselves preoccupied with past failures and mistakes or yearning for "someday" when everything will be "perfect" (whatever that means). What a waste! Your past is important because it brought you to where you are today, but it is not as important as how you see your future. That positive perception begins with being mindful. You may have heard of Brother Lawrence, who served as a cook to his fellow Carmelite monks in Paris for 60 years. Before beginning his kitchen duties, he would pray, "O my God, since Thou art with me, and I must now, in obedience to Thy commands, apply my mind to these outward things, I beseech Thee to grant me the grace to continue in Thy presence." He depended on God's Spirit to enable him to stay connected to God's presence in the midst of his work.

Another wonderful resource is HeartMath. This is an internationally recognized, non-profit research and education organization dedicated to heart-based living. You will find excellent free resources to help deal with stress and anxiety on their website as well as products and services they offer. The point is to live in the present moment and focus on your blessings and God's goodness.

I would like to share a technique I adapted from HeartMath and use personally.

I use it to release feelings such as anxiety, tension, frustration, irritation, worry and fear. This is what I do: I focus my attention on the area around my physical heart, in the center of my chest. I begin to breathe slowly and deeply but normally. I imagine my breath coming from my heart. I take a minute or two to just pay attention to my breathing and continue picturing the breath entering and exiting through the area of my heart.

As I continue my slow, relaxed heart-centered breathing, I begin to call to mind a positive feeling. I really tap into the memory and the actual feeling. I usually think about one of my children or my little grandson or even the lyrics of a worship song. For example, I picture my son, Matt's face, as he made an amazing play at first base that saved a playoff game. I see that smile and all the emotions of love flood over me. The lyrics of the song, "I Believe I Can Fly," have very special meaning to me and always evoke feelings of deep appreciation for all the Lord has done for me.

Once I feel myself experiencing those wonderful emotions, I just continue that way for a minute or two or longer if I can. I find that even doing this for a minute or two makes a huge difference and dissolves negative feelings, restoring me to a calm state where I am able to think clearly. Often I do this while tapping. Many times—I try and take a few minutes when things get very stressful—you'll be surprised at the difference—often it even changes and calms the entire atmosphere around me!

It sounds so simple, but getting yourself in what is called a state of coherence is very powerful. It's simply having heart, emotions, brainwaves and body all in harmony. We are constantly "broadcasting" with our emotions and thoughts, and as we are able to consciously stop in the midst of anxiety or upset and learn to calm ourselves, we not only improve our own health, but the environment around us as well.

Week Seven:
Putting It All Together
Integrating Soul and Spirit Practices

Spirit

Your flesh cannot overcome flesh – cravings, bad habits – only the spirit can overcome the flesh. This is part of why addressing your spirit and acknowledging its importance is so critical to long term success and true health and wholeness. You cannot just diet and ignore your spiritual health. It will not work.

Faith Confessions

Speaking faith confessions is so powerful. I do this every day and have done it for more than 30 years. Speaking them over your health and physical body is a powerful way to increase the results of your efforts to improve your health. We also know belief is very powerful. A belief is "a state or habit of mind in which trust or confidence is placed in some person or thing." Mark 9:23 says: *"Everything is possible for him who believes."* If you don't believe something is possible, for you it won't be. If you believe you will fail—you will. What you believe affects every behavior (including what you say) and every decision you make. Second Corinthians 4:13 says: *"It is written: I believed therefore I have spoken. With that same spirit of faith we also believe and therefore speak."* Couldn't have said it better myself!

Consider this equation: Fear + Doubt = limiting beliefs, which operate in your subconscious. You may be able to determine what your particular limiting beliefs are (we all have them) by asking meaningful questions. Jesus asked penetrating questions that cut to the core of a situation. Ask yourself the deep, penetrating questions. The father in Mark 9:24 expressed the idea of limiting beliefs perfectly: *"I do believe! Help me overcome my unbelief!"* (Another translation says, *"Help me overcome my doubts or weakness of faith."*)

Some examples are:

- ✓ I have no self-control/willpower;
- ✓ I have a slow metabolism;
- ✓ I love to eat;
- ✓ I hate to work out;
- ✓ I'm too stressed to take care of myself;
- ✓ I'm too old;

✓ I can never stop at one (bite/piece/cookie);

✓ It's my age/stress level/genes/hormones.

You get the idea.

The way to eliminate them is to confront them boldly:

Is this really your personal belief, or is this what you've been told by others all your life? There's a big difference there.

Ask yourself: Is this really the truth about me or about my situation? Do I really believe this? Does it benefit me?

You may not be able to determine whether this truly is your belief. One way to know is – if you consciously believe one thing – yet consistently do something else, your true belief is in conflict with what you consciously believe. That is a negative, destructive cellular memory. I mentioned above that EFT is very effective in helping to neutralize these destructive beliefs.

Replace limiting beliefs with empowering attitudes and beliefs such as:

I want to do this and I believe I can;

I can do whatever I need to with God's help because I am worth it.

Facts are subject to change. Truth is unchanging. Once you know and acknowledge the truth—you can stop believing the lie! *("You will know the truth and the truth you know and understand will make you free!"* John 8:32)

Speaking faith confessions out loud is a very effective way to accomplish this. Always speak your confessions out loud and in the present tense, as if they were accomplished fact right now, *and word them in a way that you can believe now.* That is very important because if you say something you don't believe, it will create more stress – the opposite of what you want. It may seem like a picky point—but Hebrews tells us that "*now* faith is the substance of things hoped for" and God Himself tells us He is "I AM," not I will be! Our subconscious is created to respond to our words and if we say we "will be" anything, it remains in the future somewhere.

Here are some faith-filled, health confessions you may want to adapt to your needs and include:

- ✓ "Right now I want my body to be in perfect chemical and hormonal balance and I believe it can be."
- ✓ If you can say "Right now my body *is* in perfect chemical and hormonal balance" and believe it as truth now – by all means reword the confessions that way!
- ✓ Other ways to word your confessions so that you can believe them fully now is to use the phrases "I can learn to" or "I am learning to."
- ✓ "My thyroid produces the correct amount of thyroid hormones for my body now." If that challenges you, you can say:
- ✓ "I want my thyroid to produce the correct amount of thyroid hormones for my body and I believe it does."
- ✓ "I remain within two to three pounds of my optimum weight of ___ pounds with God's help."
- ✓ "I want to remain within two to three pounds of my optimum weight of ___ pounds, and with God's help I can."
- ✓ "My belly is satisfied by the fruit of my mouth! I do not over-eat."
- ✓ "I keep my body in subjection to my spirit right now."
- ✓ "I am learning to keep my body in subjection to my spirit right now."
- ✓ "Even though all things are lawful to me, they are not all healthful and beneficial. Right now, with God's help, I break the power of any fleshly bondage, including over-eating and making unhealthy food choices."
- ✓ "Even though all things are lawful to me, they are not all healthful and beneficial. With God's help, I am learning to break the power of any fleshly bondage, including over-eating and making unhealthy food choices."
- ✓ You get the idea. Speak the confession out loud and then pay attention to how it makes you feel. If you have discomfort adjust it to something you can say with confidence. It is helpful to tap while you speak your confessions as well.

Scripture Truths

We Belong to God

Romans 12:1 NKJV: *"Present your bodies a living sacrifice, holy, acceptable to God, which is your reasonable service."*

1 Corinthians 6:19-20 NKJV: *"Do you not know that your body is the temple of the Holy Spirit who is in you, whom you have from God, and you are not your own? For you were bought at a price; therefore glorify God in your body and in your spirit, which are God's."*

In order for us to fully carry out His plans and purposes for our lives, spirit, soul and body must be strong, healthy and working together. And our bodies are not just ours alone, to treat any old way we want to. We were bought with a very high price, the Blood of Jesus. We are now stewards of these bodies and like anything else we steward, we are to glorify Him in and through them. That includes how and what we eat, think and say, whether we exercise, are physically strong and have energy or not.

You are Unique

Psalm 139:14 TLB: "*Thank you for making me so wonderfully complex! It is amazing to think about. Your workmanship is marvelous—and how well I know it.*"

Scripture tells us we are fearfully and wonderfully made! God did not make carbon copies, He created unique, one of a kind masterpieces. Our uniqueness is evident in every aspect of our lives, including what we eat. We have the responsibility and freedom to choose a way of eating and specific foods that perfectly suits us so we can fulfill God's call on our lives.

Who's the Boss?

> **1 Corinthians 6:12 NIV**: "*I have the right to do anything," you say—but not everything is beneficial. "I have the right to do anything"—but I will not be mastered by anything.*"

> **TPT**: "*It's true that our freedom allows us to do anything, but that doesn't mean that everything we do is good for us. I'm free to do as I choose, but I choose to never be enslaved to anything.*"

> **1 Corinthians 10:23 NIV**: "*I have the right to do anything, you say—but not everything is beneficial. I have the right to do anything—but not everything is constructive.*"

Our appetites, habits and choices can be beneficial or not. We can use them to improve our health or they can enslave us. This is a key verse for me. I refuse to have any master other than God.

We Are Promised Long Life

Genesis 6:3 AMPC: *"Then the Lord said, My Spirit shall not forever dwell and strive with man, for he also is flesh; but his days shall yet be 120 years."*

God intended for us to live to at least 120. Just as Moses was still strong enough to climb a mountain at 120, He meant for us to live energetic, strong, healthy, vigorous lives until the day we go home to be with Him. In order to accomplish that, we must pay attention to our spiritual health, our diet and nutrition, physical health, our thoughts and emotions. In other words, it takes addressing spirit, soul and body!

Wisdom is the Principal Thing

Proverbs 3:16 TPT: *"Wisdom extends to you long life in one hand and wealth and promotion in the other."*

Proverbs 4:10 NLT: *"My child, listen to me and do as I say, and you will have a
long, good life."*

Proverbs 3:2 NKJV: *"For length of days and long life, and peace they will add to you."*

Proverbs 9:11 AMPC: *"For by me [Wisdom from God] your days shall be multiplied, and the years of your life shall be increased."*

Using wisdom in every facet of your life will only bring good to you. Where your health is concerned, wisdom is the key to length of days.

Trusting God Brings Health

Proverbs 3:8 NKJV: *"It will be health to your flesh, and strength to your bones."*

Your Heart Keeps You Healthy

Proverbs 17:22 TPT: *"A joyful, cheerful heart brings healing to both body and soul. But the one whose heart is crushed struggles with sickness and depression."*

Your spiritual heart, as I said before, is a combination of your spirit and soul. It is your innermost being. God breathed the breath of life into Adam which imparted His spirit into him, and he became a living soul. Therefore, it impacts your entire being – spirit, soul and body. Keeping your heart clean, clear of offense and bitterness and full of peace and faith brings joy. If depression and sadness are always issues, perhaps you need to do a heart check.

> **Proverbs 4:23 TPT**: *"So above all, guard the affections of your heart, for they affect all that you are. Pay attention to the welfare of your innermost being, for from there flows the wellspring of life."*

Keeping your heart established and secure on the Word of God is the best medicine for health and long life.

> **Proverbs 14:30 TPT**: *"A tender, tranquil heart will make you healthy, but jealousy*
> *can make you sick."*

> **AMPC**: *"A calm and undisturbed mind and heart are the life and health of the body, but envy, jealousy, and wrath are like rottenness of the bones."*

Weak bones, arthritis and all kinds of other problems related to bone health are linked to a heart not free from envy, jealousy and wrath.

Keep it Real

> **Proverbs 23:1-3 NKJV**: *"When you sit down to eat with a ruler, consider carefully what is before you; And put a knife to your throat, if you are a man given to appetite. Do not desire his delicacies, for they are deceptive food.*

So many "foods" on the grocery store shelves are "deceptive foods." They are not truly foods at all, but they are food-like products. Another translation calls them "deceitful meat".

Bottom Line

> **1 Corinthians 10:31 NLT**: *"So whether you eat or drink, or whatever you do, do it all for the glory of God."*

Soul:

The main soul issue is to develop positive habits and thinking in the area of food and exercise. As I have said, your subconscious mind is very powerful and in order to change your body, you have to reprogram your thinking.

Releasing weight and getting fit, once and for all, boils down to three basic concepts:

First you must honestly acknowledge the root cause—*why are you overweight?*

- ✓ Is it a discipline "deficiency"? Consistently choosing wrong foods?
- ✓ A lack of solid information?
- ✓ Simply eating too much and moving too little?
- ✓ Laziness?
- ✓ Fear?
- ✓ Do you have no idea why you seem to continually sabotage yourself?

Next, you have to change *how* you think about it. Once you understand what your particular "root" is, you must think about it in a different way. Thinking the same thoughts will cause you to produce the same results, so you must change your thinking.

Finally, you must commit to a realistic plan and take action in order to arrive at the result you desire. This is what you have been doing these last seven weeks!

It's really very simple: every condition can be traced back to one or more "roots." A true solution reveals and addresses the root(s), not just symptoms. Being overweight is a symptom. You must always look past the symptom to deal with the root. Treating symptoms alone is like constantly putting out fires!

This is why I offer resources like my coaching and EFT – getting to the root is the ONLY way to resolve any issue once and for all.

Your attitude or perception is the personal lens through which you view life. Shifting your thinking can make all the difference in creating a different future. You can change your attitude by learning to refocus your lens. Change what you think and speak and you will change your emotions and behavior. When you change the way you look at things, the things you look at change. The Bible tells us our words are powerful—life and death are in the power of your tongue (Proverbs 18:21).

Thoughts about refocusing your lens:

- ✓ Problems can become challenges;

- ✓ "failure," is simply a new lesson to learn;
- ✓ frustration becomes fulfillment;
- ✓ chaos becomes order;
- ✓ rules become routines;
- ✓ older means wiser (I especially like this one!);
- ✓ confusion becomes clarity;
- ✓ plateaus are transitions—time to revisit and revise your routines;
- ✓ you don't "have" to exercise (or do anything!), you *choose* to;
- ✓ a "diet" is temporary; a nutrition and fitness plan like this is a "blueprint" for new, health-building habits;
  - ✓ I "can't" means you don't want to, choose not to or are not ready to – yet. It short circuits your subconscious from coming up with solutions.
  - ✓ Why not imagine possibilities and think instead: "What could I do?"
  - ✓ Use the word "could" today on your behalf!
  - ✓ What "could" you do today to eat better?
  - ✓ What "could" you do to get more activity in your day?
  - ✓ What "could" you do to keep your thinking positive and inspired?

"Could" is a powerful way to keep yourself moving forward toward success in releasing weight and getting fit! It puts you in the driver's seat, so to speak, and it's always good to be working from a place of strength and control.

Words can make all the difference in your success. Research shows that when tempted to eat a treat you really don't want to or when a craving strikes, saying, **"I *Don't* Eat That"** instead of **"I *can't* eat that"** helped 80% of women stick to their meal plans! "Can't" implies something you want is being withheld from you. Saying instead, "I Don't" or "I Choose Not To" is empowering - you make the choice! Watch what you say. Your body is always listening!

Excuses are total dead-ends! Are any of these excuses keeping you in bondage? Refocusing smashes those excuses and the bondages they previously held you in and creates new freedom. Look at how refocusing changes them:

"Dieting is too hard (or boring, restrictive)." You need to make a firm commitment; prioritize properly and simplify by creating routines.

"I can't live without (fill in the specific food or foods)." You don't have to! You can still visit those "old friends," just not as often! Get to know some new, healthier "friends" you will like even better!

"No one in my family can ever lose weight." Nutrition, habits and lifestyle account for 80% of any physical condition—genetics only 20%. Neither your past nor your genes need define your future.

"It's no fun if I can't have (fill in the blank)." Life won't be much fun if you don't take care of your health. Balance and moderation are the keys.

"I have too many responsibilities (caring for my family, a demanding job)." You must take care of yourself first in order to take care of anyone else. Scripture tells us we are to love our neighbor (that includes family!) as we (first) love ourselves! (Romans 13:9)

"But I love eating out!" Once you learn how to make healthier choices and develop your self-discipline "muscle," you can eat wherever you like.

Finally, activate your emotions, both positive and negative, to find your compelling "why." Think carefully about what the most emotional, life-changing, rewarding reason to stay with the plan is. Feel that emotion deeply. Is it to set a great example for your children; to make your spouse or children proud of you; to be more active; lower blood sugar; to feel great about yourself; to avoid having to take pharmaceutical drugs; remain strong and active; whatever it is, it must touch your emotions powerfully.

Then imagine the most emotional, painful reason—whatever provokes feelings of disappointment, shame—for instance, your child struggling with the same issue down the road because of your example; being unable to fulfill your life goals; becoming sick and unable to care for yourself. I am suggesting you use the emotions God gave us to your advantage.

When you can clearly feel the positive and negative, and you have an important, concrete, compelling "WHY" for wanting to achieve your goal, studies show you are MUCH more likely to stay consistent and succeed. In fact, once you are clear about this, write a descriptive statement of each emotion that you can go back to and read in order to activate those emotions. Using the picture visualization is also powerful here.

Detoxing Emotions Trapped in your Cells

Some experts have done research revealing that negative emotions can actually become trapped in your cells. If you find yourself reacting to a situation with an emotional response that is far more severe than that situation warrants, then this may be a clue that you are dealing with stored negative emotions from your past, also referred to as destructive cellular memories.

So why would negative emotions become trapped in your cells? It's usually because you didn't know how to deal with them in the first place. This would especially be true of emotions from childhood. In fact, one doctor has found from years of research and experience that most people are more affected by their past than they are by their present circumstances. That's a very important point I don't want to gloss over. The Bible clearly tells us "faith is now" and God Himself says He is "I AM"—all present-tense. When we constantly live stuck in our emotional past, we are not in touch with and aware of present spiritual reality and what God desires to do in our "today."

Negative emotions can become trapped and stuck anywhere in your body. For example, according to Chinese medicine, resentment is an emotion associated with the gallbladder. The gallbladder meridian is found at the shoulders. Tension in the shoulders could signify a toxic gallbladder and suppressed resentment.

When you do a detox or fast, weak, dead and dying cells (which carry trapped emotions) are rapidly released from your body. So, besides physically detoxifying your body, you can release those trapped emotions as well. Staying adequately hydrated helps you to more efficiently process emotions as well!

Your liver is your primary detoxification organ as I said previously. If it is unable to remove a toxin, it will actually store it in an effort to keep it from circulating in your blood. This is why many people's livers have become toxic storage containers.

In Chinese medicine, most organs are connected to a specific emotion, and your liver is the organ connected to anger. A toxic liver is said to lead to problems controlling or letting go of anger. The more toxic the habits and the longer the problem exists, the worse the situation becomes. Extremely toxic habits would include smoking, taking drugs, being exposed to pesticides, as well as regularly eating junk, chemically laden, processed or genetically modified foods.

Anger itself is simply an emotion. It is not good or bad, and like all emotions, should never be suppressed. Emotions that are suppressed remain in the body way past their time and they always come out eventually—usually at the worst possible time and in the worst possible way.

So, the condition of your liver can actually determine how you experience and express anger. When your liver is toxic, you'll feel anger longer, more intensely, more passionately, and have a more difficult time letting it go. It can become an overwhelming, overpowering emotion that devastates your life.

Your emotions have a strong and direct connection to the state of your physical health. The condition and health of your liver powerfully affects how you feel and how you experience anger, which naturally then affects how you act and react to situations or people who trigger it. A toxic liver could be an underlying cause of expressing anger in a destructive, inappropriate manner!

So, if you find you are experiencing "anger management" problems, consider the fact that a toxic liver could be an underlying cause and take steps to detoxify yourself. Effective herbs for liver cleansing are dandelion root, burdock, milk thistle, and licorice root. Overnight from 11 pm until 3 am the energy is strongest in the gall bladder and liver, so taking liver herbs right before bed can help support this function.

Also, according to Chinese Medicine, digestion is naturally slower in the evening as the energy is weakest in those meridians at that time. Food stays in the stomach and tends to ferment, leading to gas, bloating, reflux and discomfort. Energy is drawn from other organs to help digest food. These organs cleanse the blood and control sleep. They become taxed when we eat late at night. We get indigestion, insomnia and a feeling of not being well rested in the morning. Eating late at night strains our liver, drawing energy from it to help us digest food. This is why I recommend you stop eating by 7 pm.

WHERE DO WE GO FROM HERE?

Incorporating Principles

I wanted to reiterate that you should consider this to be a blueprint you can adapt in any way that works best for you. Incorporate the principles that make sense for your goals and needs and fit most readily with your unique personality and into your lifestyle. If it's too hard—you won't do it, plain and simple. I suggest incorporating principles because sometimes there will be one area that works really well for you and another that doesn't, in any plan, no matter how good! I believe that to be true of many things. Kenneth Hagin once said: "Eat the hay and spit out the sticks"—or something similar. That is the best advice I can give you—take whatever you can use and what works for you and discard what doesn't. That is also why I help clients adjust the plan to their needs when we work together in coaching.

This plan has been forged from trial and error, over 30 years of personal experience, questioning experts and voracious reading of any information I could get my hands on concerning fitness, weight loss and natural health. While I have never been extremely overweight, in my early 40s I gained about 15 lbs. even though I was careful with my diet and exercised every day. That was the inspiration and impetus for me to create this plan. By incorporating these principles I was able to lose the weight and have kept it off for more than 20 years.

Over the years I have read and studied many "diets" and plans, tried them with varying degrees of success and have done exactly what I suggest you do—I have adapted principles that I found to fit my health philosophy and lifestyle from each. I began by saying there are hundreds of diets out there and we all know there's pretty much nothing new under the sun! (Ecclesiastes 1:9)

<u>The core of this program is getting back to basics, eating the best quality, one-ingredient, whole foods in a form as close to how God created them and honoring your body as the temple of the Holy Spirit.</u>

90/10 Rule

Once you finish the seven weeks, you can incorporate what I call "treat" days as I already mentioned. Other plans refer to them as "cheat" days. You can call them whatever you are comfortable with as long as it doesn't cause negative thoughts or emotions. You do not have to strictly watch everything you eat 100% of the time. Life is to be enjoyed and favorite foods are part of that enjoyment! If you are careful 80-90% of the time, what you eat the other 10-20% of the time will not have that great an impact.

I always say, it is not what you do between Thanksgiving and New Year's (within reason!) that matters, but what you do between New Year's and Thanksgiving. If you constantly deprive yourself of foods you love, forbidding yourself to ever have them, you will begin to crave them more and more, constantly think about them and, finally, you will lose all control. That's not what you want. You want to be in control of your choices, and you can choose to have a treat day every week or two.

This way, any cravings you might have are satisfied and you can get right back onto your clean way of eating while doing no damage to your overall progress. This is why I suggest looking at this plan as a flexible blueprint that you can adjust to your needs, rather than a rigid "all or nothing" diet. Being flexible allows you to bend. If you are rigid, you are in danger of snapping and breaking!

Excuses, Perception, Genes and Victim Mentality

"I 'inherited' my mother's temper/tendency to gain weight/fat thighs/voracious appetite/negative attitude/lack of self-control." If any of these excuses sound familiar, chances are you're playing the "genes" card! It's very easy to look at your family history and decide that whatever health issue you are dealing with is genetic and there's little you can do about it.

We all have certain specific genetic predispositions. For example, you may have a genetic predisposition toward diabetes, obesity, heart problems or cancer. I am not denying that your family history may predispose you to certain diseases. All of my grandparents except for one, most of my aunts and uncles and my mother ALL died from cancer. Does it seem to run in my family? Gallop may be more like it. I acknowledge the history, but I do not believe it destines me or my children to go down the same path.

Consider a different question—what really runs in your family, genes or habits? Research confirms that although heredity and familial disposition toward certain conditions have an effect on physical health, it only accounts for approximately 20%—lifestyle and nutrition account for close to 80%! This tells me that while we can acknowledge our family's health history and be aware of it, we need not repeat it. Rather than just continue to perpetuate the habits we may have grown up with, we have the power to choose to change them and improve the outcome. (There's that word "choose" again!)

When you choose to believe a problem is genetic or you just inherited it—you are saying it cannot be changed, you are doomed to be this way and there's NOTHING you can do about it! You make yourself a victim and relinquish responsibility for your thoughts, beliefs and actions. It's been scientifically proven that your perception of a situation or condition (how you see it) matters more than the condition itself. What you think and believe is so powerful—it can change your DNA!

While changing lifelong habits may not be easy, remember, your choices not only affect you, but future generations as well. We need not feel we're doomed to suffer from the same problems and diseases as our parents and grandparents. Deuteronomy 30:19 encourages us to choose life, for ourselves and for our children. We can choose to do things differently. Our parents did the best they knew to do. Since we know better, we must make the choice to do better.

We must also embrace the truth that as Christians we now have a different, better Bloodline, one in which there is no disease! By doing these things we can change our old perceptions and create a new "history," passing down vibrant health, wholeness and faith for generations to come.

Tweaking the Plan Moving Forward

Whether you achieved your goal in these seven weeks or still have a ways to go, you may want to incorporate some "tweaks" to the basic plan just to change things up. So I offer these two strategies you can try.

Progression Principle

I've read research by Dr. George L. Blackburn about changing your "set point." I've adapted this into my own progressive approach to releasing weight that can help you avoid plateaus. Here's how it works:

Commit to this program for the seven weeks. If you reached your weight loss goal within that time, you can then transition to the maintenance plan (just be very careful not to gain weight but to maintain what you've lost.)

*If you have not yet reached your goal, you can remain on the plan until you have reached your goal before switching to the maintenance plan, or you can go on the maintenance plan for two to three weeks now and then get back on the basic plan.

After two or three weeks on the maintenance plan, assuming you have more weight to lose, return to the plan (at Week Three, limiting healthy whole grains and starchy carbs to one meal early in the day or Weeks One and Two, without any grains or starchy carbs) for another four weeks and then re-evaluate your progress. Dr. Blackburn found the maintenance period gives your body and mind time to adjust to your new weight. He found people went on to lose an additional 10% of their body weight more quickly and easily. This has worked really well for me and for some clients.

It's a strategy you may want to try.

Carb Cycling

Another strategy you might find helpful is my simplified way to use "carb cycling" when you need to break through a plateau, drop a few pounds or just want to give your metabolism a boost.

Carb cycling is simply alternating your meal plans between the no starchy carb days from weeks one and two, your basic plan from weeks three and up where you eat specific, healthy whole grains and starchy carbs, in moderation and only at breakfast or lunch, and finally the "high carb" day where you add extra carbs. You are still eating the same clean, fresh, whole, nutrient-dense foods—the basic plan never changes. This is simply one way to "tweak" it when you need to—for instance, before or after vacation or holidays.

Here are the basic rules:

Keep your protein consumption stable—do not decrease it. Be sure to have your four to six ounces of protein at each meal as you have been.

Continue taking your fiber supplement, your raw salad and plenty of fibrous green vegetables in your meals. Adequate fiber is critical.

Be sure to drink the proper amount of water for your weight and the right amount of salt.

No Carb Days: Serving of protein at each meal; unlimited non-starchy vegetables; two pieces of fruit; two to four tablespoons of healthy fat.

*Do your weight training on your no carb days since you can add an extra whey protein shake. Be sure to eat enough. Don't allow yourself to fall below 1,000 calories—hence the extra fat allowed.

Maintenance (Basic Plan) Days: Protein at each meal; unlimited non-starchy vegetables; two pieces of fruit; two tablespoons of healthy fat and *one serving* of healthy whole grain or starchy carb at breakfast **or** lunch (see the list from Week Three for healthy carbs to add.)

High Carb Day: Follow the basic plan, adding a serving of healthy carb at breakfast, lunch *and* dinner. This should add approximately 500 calories of healthy carb.

*Do your long cardio or high intensity interval training on these high carb days.

Cycle for a week or two using a schedule like this:

- ✓ Monday: No Carb
- ✓ Tuesday: Maintenance
- ✓ Wednesday: High Carb
- ✓ Thursday: No Carb
- ✓ Friday: Maintenance
- ✓ Saturday: High Carb
- ✓ Sunday: Maintenance

Weekly Detox Day

I like to take my supplements for six days of the week and have one day off with no supplements. I believe your body responds better when you give it a day off and it follows along with having a Sabbath day of rest.

That being said, I usually make Sunday my supplement free day. When I am having a treat day, I do it separate from my supplement free day.

I like to take advantage of not having my daily supplements and instead have a few activated charcoal capsules or clay capsules. I still drink all my water, and taking either of these supplements helps absorb any toxins without interfering with any of my supplements.

I like Red Desert Clay and use it for oral health and even as a face mask, but in this instance, I purchased some empty vegetarian capsules that I fill myself with the clay and usually take four of them and two activated charcoal capsules with at least 16 ounces of water. I make sure I have at least 16-32 more ounces of water throughout the day as well.

Both the clay and activated charcoal are known to absorb (soak up) as well as adsorb (attract like a magnet attracts metal) certain toxins. I can't stress enough the importance of drinking adequate water when doing this. Without enough water, either of these substances can cause constipation and the whole point of using them to detoxify is to flush the toxins out of the body. So do this on a day when you are able to drink enough water comfortably.

What Do You Believe and Expect?

Mark 11:23 clearly tells us if we believe that the words we say shall come to pass and not doubt in our hearts, we will have whatever we say. Jesus Himself tells us in Matthew 21:22, *"And whatever things you ask in prayer, believing, you will receive."* These scriptures are clear and as Christians we know God cannot and does not lie, so what He has said is truth. However, we may not have been able to experience it in this way in our own lives. The main thrust of these scriptures is faith, belief and expectation.

Belief and expectation are powerful spiritual forces that go hand in hand, affecting every area of our lives. It isn't hard to believe that expectation is a powerful thing. The more you believe you're going to benefit from anything—a treatment, a procedure—the more likely it is that you will experience a benefit from it. It is sometimes called the Placebo Effect, but it all comes down to belief and expectation.

Let's apply that to this fitness plan. The more you believe that putting the proper fuel in your body, keeping yourself cleansed spirit, soul and body, exercising and learning better habits will improve your health and body, the more consistently you will do them and the more effective those actions will be.

Begin by thinking about and writing in your log what your specific beliefs are about health and fitness. Keep in mind that your behavior is the truest test of what you really believe. For example, do you believe:

- ✓ "Exercising is hard?"
- ✓ "Exercise won't change your body?"
- ✓ "You hate vegetables?"
- ✓ "You could never give up sugar?"

- ✓ "You will always be overweight no matter what you do?"
- ✓ "You don't like "healthy" food? It doesn't matter what you eat—it all goes to fat anyway?"

Be honest – there's no condemnation here. You can't address what you don't honestly acknowledge.

Now write down what you truly expect:

- ✓ Do you expect this plan to be hard?
- ✓ Do you expect eating this way to be tasteless or boring?
- ✓ Do you really expect to reach your goal?
- ✓ Do you expect to be too tired to exercise regularly?

Again, be very honest.

Now ask yourself these questions:

- ✓ Is what you believe and truly expect sabotaging your progress?
- ✓ Do you really want to change what is limiting you so you can succeed?

If you really don't or are not ready to—be honest with yourself, or else you will just keep sabotaging your own efforts and end up frustrated and discouraged.

That last question is the bottom line to truly rebooting your fitness beliefs. Recommit yourself to eliminating those beliefs that are limiting your progress. Your beliefs and expectations are such powerful forces—you must have them working for you and not against you—even subconsciously!

Success!

I want to congratulate you if you have gone through this seven week plan step-by-step and reached your goal. That's an awesome accomplishment! Many people need the accountability and support of a coach, and that is why I offer this program both ways—including the coaching component and as a book that people can do at their own pace, privately. You can find out more about the seven week coaching plan on my website or visit the resource page here: http://www.threedimensionalvitality.com/resource-page-for-book.html or https://bit.ly/2Eqo1sb

Please contact me at ann@threedimensionalvitality.com and tell me your story. I want to share your results so that others may be encouraged by them, and I know they will be! Feel free to share any comments you have about the plan as well. I am always trying to improve it, and client feed-back is very valuable to me.

I also invite you to visit my website and sign up for the free newsletter and other resources.

I just want to take a moment to talk about guarantees. I would never claim that everyone who uses this program will reach their goal. There are no guarantees simply because you are in control of how well you implement the plan. Even when I coach clients, I cannot "make" them to do what they need to, *so the only one who can guarantee your success is you.*

From experience working with many different types of people, no matter how well something works and how balanced it is, there will always be a few people who don't get the results they wished for—even if they followed it to the best of their ability. This has to do with issues unique to that individual. That is why this plan includes spirit and soul. Without those aspects being addressed, you may lose weight initially, but you will eventually end up right back where you started. That's also why you are encouraged to run this by your personal physician or health care practitioner. There may be underlying issues that must be addressed first. Finally, that is why I recommend you consider it a blueprint and incorporate those principles that work best for you.

Every client who has used this plan and made the commitment to follow it to the best of their ability for the seven weeks or longer has gotten excellent results. I developed this plan originally for myself and this is how I eat and live every day of my life, over 20 years later!

Once again, I congratulate you and look forward to hearing your success story!

BONUS

As a bonus and my gift to you, I am including:

31 Day devotional, Daily Tips for Wholeness. Just go to this page on my website: http://www.threedimensionalvitality.com/daily-tips-for-wholeness.html or https://bit.ly/2GBTOfG and put your email address in the box. You will begin receiving the emails as soon as you follow the instructions in the confirmation email. I hope they bless and encourage you!

There are numerous free resources I make available,, including the 15-minute consultation, 15-minute Tapping Session, weekly No-Nonsense Nutrition Report, my blog, recipes, interviews and podcasts.

Just go to http://www.threedimensionalvitality.com or http://www.annmusico.com.

Remember, you can access information for any of the resources mentioned in the book on the Resource page here:

http://www.threedimensionalvitality.com/resource-page-for-book.html or https://bit.ly/2Eqo1sb

I sincerely invite you to visit, get to know me and what I do better, and share your thoughts with me. I love hearing from you and I answer all emails.

Wishing you health, wholeness and blessings,

Ann

About The Author

Ann Musico is a certified holistic health coach, author, wellness blogger and independent nutritional consultant who has worked with women of all ages to empower them to exemplify lives of vibrant health and wholeness – spirit, soul and body – in a way that is simple and effective. She received her certification from Jordan Rubin's Biblical Health Institute and is the founder of the Three Dimensional Vitality website.

Her focus is on nutrition, detox and healthy, long term weight loss because she believes those areas are most often the root cause of so many other problems. She addresses them not only from the physical but from the spirit and soul as well, which are often overlooked. She offers numerous coaching options as well as free resources, which you can find at her website http://www.threedimensionalvitality.com. You can learn more about her on her Learn About Me page.

Ok, that's the formal introduction to who I am and why you should listen to what I say about nutrition or weight loss, but I want to tell you why helping women get and stay healthy is my passion.

First of all my relationship with my Lord Jesus Christ is the foundation of my life and of everything I do.

I am a wife of 35 years at the time this book is being published and the proud mother of three amazing adult children. All I ever wanted to do in life was to be a good mom and God gave me that incredible opportunity and privilege. While no one does that perfectly, including me, I am grateful to say I have three healthy, loving, talented, successful, wonderful children who love the Lord and are building healthy, loving families of their own. I could never ask for more!

My mother had many emotional and physical issues and passed away very suddenly just before I met my husband. So she never met him, wasn't at our wedding, never got to see and enjoy my children, her grandchildren, or be a part of their lives. I wanted to create a different legacy. My mother died at the same age I am the day I am writing this, and sadly she missed so much.

I know how great it feels to be strong and fit and able to keep up with my children and now my grandchildren. I want that to be every woman's reality. I want every woman to have the opportunity and ability to look and feel her best and to enjoy her life to the fullest. I believe we women are the gatekeepers and influencers of the next generation and we have a responsibility and the privilege of helping our families to live healthier lives by setting the example.

This is the core of my mission and what drives me every day.

www.ingramcontent.com/pod-product-compliance
Lightning Source LLC
Chambersburg PA
CBHW081655270326
41933CB00017B/3173